Wild WORKOUT POWERFLEX

Bring Out the Animal in You

The **FORYSTEKS'**

LU Books
A Division of Liberty University Press

www.TheWildWorkout.com

Wild WORKOUT POWERFLEX

ISBN: 978-1-935986-07-2 Paperback

Published by:

LU Books

LU Books
A Division of Liberty University Press
1971 University Blvd.
Lynchburg, VA 24551
www.liberty.edu/libertyuniversitypress

Cover Wrap Design by:
Megan Johnson

Interior Design and Layout by:
Heather Kirk

www.TheWildWorkout.com

NOTE: The exercises and advice contained within this book may be too strenuous and dangerous for some people, and the reader should consult their health practitioner before engaging in them. The information in this book is for educational purposes only. Neither the publisher nor author is engaged in rendering professional advice or services to the individual reader. All matters regarding physical and mental health should be supervised by a health practitioner knowledgeable in treating that particular condition. Neither the author nor the publisher shall be liable or responsible for any loss, injury, or damage allegedly arising from any information or suggestion in this book.

TABLE OF CONTENTS

FOREWORD

by Kabeer Gbaja-Biamila

Looking back at my 9 years playing for the Green Bay Packers, 4 years of college football at San Diego State, 4 years of football at Crenshaw High School and even a few years of organized football before that, I can't recall when sports, fitness and physical strength has not been a part of my life. Staying fit and strong was never an issue for me as I had football, weight training, and other forms of physical conditioning at my beckon call (Actually, the call of my coaches is more like it!) I don't remember the last time I didn't have access to a training facility or someone instructing me on what exercises to do, that is, until my last season in the NFL two years ago. I didn't realize how spoiled and dependent I was on my coaches and the training facilities to keep me "in shape" until they were no longer available.

After that I found I was making excuses for getting out of my top physical condition — no time, no trainer, no facility, no working out at all! I started to think that the only way for me to get back into shape was if I decided to play for the NFL again, and if not, it was downhill for me. God, however, showed me different. In 2 Peter 1:3 God says that He "has given us everything we need for life and godliness" — including everything we need to stay fit and strong; no gym or trainer required! It was then that God introduced me to Jim Forystek and the PowerFlex program. I was intrigued at how physically fit he and his whole family were, without the use of weight machines or hours spent at the gym. He also explained to me how naturally strong God made the beasts He created, and that He has given me the ability to maintain my strength as well. I was amazed to learn about the various movements of these magnificent animals and how incorporating those same movements can help me stay strong. Even the NFL acknowledges the power, flexibility, and agility of God's creatures, (ie... the Panthers, Rams, Jaguars, Bears, Lions, etc.)

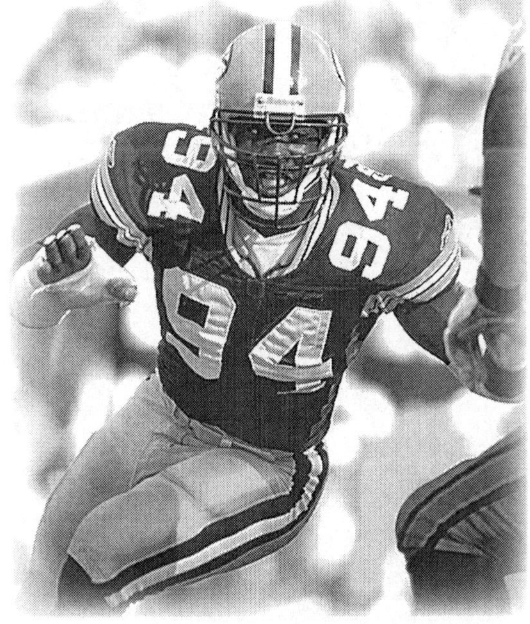

The great thing about PowerFlex is that I can conveniently fit this program into my busy schedule, perform these exercises in the comfort of my own home, and have my wife and children partake in a workout regimen with me! I also don't have to worry about the jarring and strain on my joints like before. Not only am I saving my body unnecessary pain, with PowerFlex all parts of my body are being utilized, not just the ones targeted for football. No more muscle imbalance, heavy weights and unnatural weight lifting exercises! With PowerFlex, I have no excuse!

The Bible also says, "Let not the mighty man boast in his might, nor let the wise man boast in his wisdom, ...but let he who boasts, boast in the Lord." After getting to know Jim Forystek and his family, it is evident that he is a man of God who is not relying on his own knowledge or strength but truly seeks God for everything, including the PowerFlex program. God is the creator of our human body and He knows exactly how it works and how to keep it at its best. With that as the Forystek foundation, you can trust that PowerFlex will be a great tool for you to get in shape and stay that way.

His Servant,

Jesus! #94

Kabeer Gbaja-Biamila

ACKNOWLEDGEMENTS

from Jimmy Forystek

Health and Fitness can be broken down into two parts: The first is getting fit, and the second is STAYING fit! Along the way it is very helpful and motivating to have other people help you along your way to achieve your lifelong health and fitness goals!

I would personally like to thank my dad for creating the Wild Workout® PowerFlex® exercise program, because it is and always will be my source for health, strength, flexibility, and muscle definition. He has been such a motivational influence for health and fitness in my life. Starting back from when I was just a young boy, I always saw my dad doing interesting movements, though I didn't know what they were at the time, they always looked like a lot of fun. He explained to me how they were called exercises and they helped to build your muscles and body strong and healthy. As a young boy, or even an old boy for that matter, who doesn't want to have big, strong muscles?

My dad always encouraged me to be active and would always let me exercise with him teaching me his exercises. I remember when I was in eighth grade I worked hard with the Wild Workout® Power-Flex® abdominal exercises and in little time the exercises paid off and gave me a nicely defined "6-pack." My abdominal muscles were the first targeted muscle group I became very satisfied with. As I stated before exercise has two parts getting fit, and STAYING fit. I remember particularly one evening not too long after my abs became strong and very defined, my dad said, "Jimmy you really have great abs, now how about targeting another muscle group to get another area developed as much as you would like?" I agreed, and he helped me perfect and perform the chest exercises and I soon started noticing my chest and upper body becoming more defined and growing.

I really got into doing the entire program (all 9 sections) seriously when I entered high school. I was now going to be playing sports and I wanted to be the best athlete I could. I was still young with my body developing and growing and it was so great to have such a joint-friendly, effective program that wasn't going to compress my spine, hurt my joints, or cause unnecessary injury. I loved the fast, effective results I obtained from the exercises. Wild Workout® Powerflex® made the initial getting fit part quite easy (with some hard work of course). I specifically went through the program targeting all major muscle groups plus the Spine section, and Speed, Energy and Endurance section, and thank my dad for always being an example and teaching me the dynamic, powerful, yet safe and healthy way to exercise for a TOTAL BODY WORKOUT head-to-toe!

I also would like to thank my two brothers, John and Jed for always being there to workout with me and encouragement me. There are always going to be days where you don't feel like exercising but it is those days where other people can give you the encouragement and energy you need. Whether it was performing the Chest, Abs, Legs, Arms, Shoulders, Neck, Spine, Back or Speed Energy and Endurance exercises, my family was always an encouragement to me because they made health and fitness a priority in their life. They also cared enough about the others around them to help them when they needed it, including me. I remember days when I was doing my training for football performing the Speed, Energy and Endurance section, my brother Jed, who was a lot younger at the time, yet still wanted to give me a good challenge, so he would ride his bike against me. As my brothers got older and faster, we would always push each other to be better, faster, and the best we could be while still having fun and making exercise ENJOYABLE! I always had a blast and it made me the athlete I wanted to be, while giving me the physique and performance I desired. After high school I had the privilege to play 4 years of Division 1-FCS college football at Liberty University where we finished my final season in 2007 Big South Champions for the first time in school history.

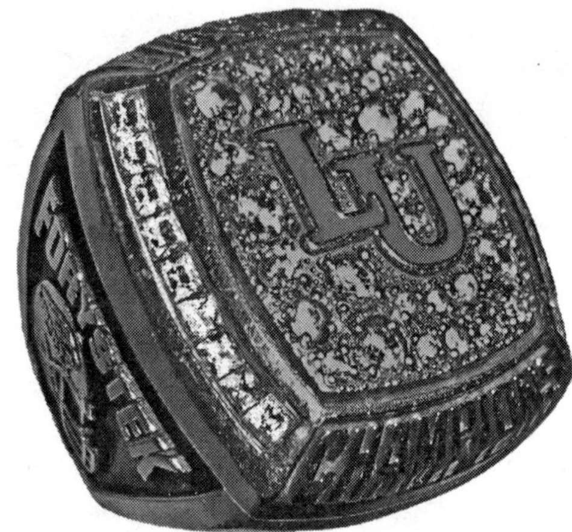

Lastly, I would like to thank my Grandpa and all the people along the way who were an inspiration and encouragement to my dad on his health and fitness journey, because it was my dad who gave me the tools and exercises necessary to embark on the journey of my own!

I know one day the Lord Jesus is coming to bring me home. He will give me a glorified body that makes Superman's look sick, one that will fly with the angels, walk on the Crystal Sea, and stroll down the streets of gold. Until then He has given me this earthly body, that when kept in shape, and is fit and healthy, it can do absolutely amazing, fantastic things that will blow your mind at any age! Jesus for the spirit and Wild Workout® for the body! WOW! You too can know eternal life and a glorified body is yours if you put your faith and trust in Jesus, being fit for eternity, now that's the way to go!

It does not matter what age anyone currently is, exercise does wonders for the body! I have always and will always continue to use Wild Workout® Powerflex® because it is the program I can use the REST of my life. It is a program that doesn't require machines, equipment, weights, or dumbbells. It will not put the unnecessary stress and pressure on my joints that so many other programs so often do. If you are a young teenager, a wise 80 year old, or someone in between, Wild Workout® Powerflex® is the program for you and you truly can make it your lifetime program just as I have done and I thank my dad for developing the program and all of my family for being such an encouragement.

Amongst the Forysteks' this truly is a workout passed on from generation to generation and we are greatly pleased to be able to pass this tradition on to you through Wild Workout® PowerFlex®. So please when you need that motivation, that inspiration, and the encouragement to never give up look to us because we are here to help, strengthen, and encourage you on your path to lifelong health and fitness.

For Health and Fitness,

Jimmy Forystek

---

from John Forystek

Growing up I would always watch my Dad doing his work out; Panther Flexes, Dolphin Flexes, Eagle Flexes etc... and I always wanted to be just like dad. I would look forward to when my dad was getting ready to work out because I would always go along side him and mimic his movements. It was always exciting when he would show me the natural way to build our bodies just like the animals. I would then mimic the movements of the ferocious Panther, the powerful Gorilla, the fearless Shark and it was just an enjoyable time that I would get to spend with my dad. He would encourage me, help me and make it fun to workout with me and the whole family!

He also showed me how to develop each area of the body specifically for what task I had ahead of me. After getting me involved in music and playing the drums, my dad helped me develop my muscles to play with quickness, speed, agility, and dexterity to excel above the competition which later on earned me numerous gold medals and awards. I thank God for blessing me with my dad who led the way to a strong healthy life, and equipped me with the tools that I needed to succeed.

I also want to thank Him for blessing me with two great brothers Jimmy and Jed. I am the middle boy, which means I always had either my older stronger brother Jimmy or younger brother Jed around to work out with, rough house with, and wrestle with to shape my character. We would always encourage each other to be their best, and be around to workout with on days when you just didn't feel like it. I remember the cold Wisconsin winters when we would decide to finish our Camel trots and Cheetah dashes in sometimes negative temperatures. We would bundle up from head to toe leaving only our eyes exposed then make our way to the park where twice around the block equaled a mile.

By the time we were finished we were covered in frost and had icicles hanging from our eyelashes but it sure was a fun time working out with my brothers and knowing I always had someone right there beside me. No matter if it was training for football, body building, tennis, or just a good hard workout we always had a training partner and I thank God for that.

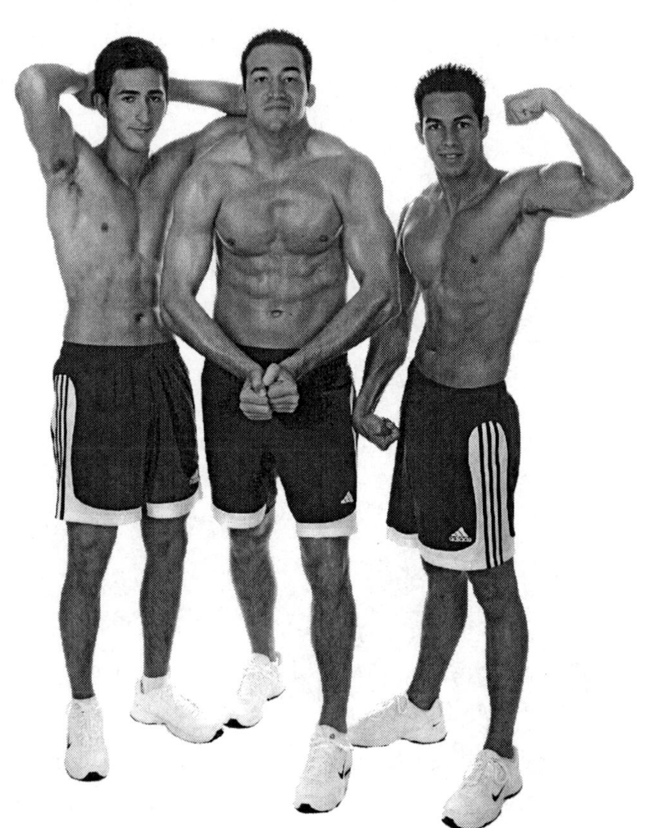

I know that you are on your way to a lifetime of health and fitness since you choose the Wild Workout® program and I wish you the best. This program is all that you will need to get a great body and excel above the competition! Just as it has worked for so many others, you now will have your own success story to tell. Remember to be consistent in your PowerFlexes and keep your eyes on the goal it is not very far off, you just have to reach out and take it!

Your Friend,

John Forystek

John Forystek

INTRODUCTION

Your body is the most AWESOME invention God ever came up with! It builds itself, heals itself, repairs itself, and has a built-in heating and cooling system, an electrical power plant bursting with energy, a built-in defense system, and a central processing unit in the human brain that puts any computer to shame. Plus your body was designed to last a *long* time and feel good and healthy while being alive—the key is not just to add more years to your life but to add more life to your years! It is one of the only things in the universe that gets better the more you use it! Wow! It is truly awesome!

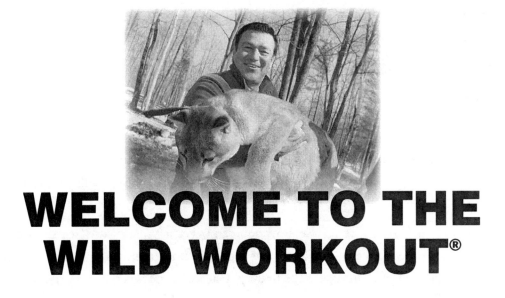

WELCOME TO THE WILD WORKOUT®

Thank you for choosing Wild Workout® PowerFlex®, the total body workout program. Make no mistake: Wild Workout® gives real results that will blow you away, and results without the use of steroids, drugs, weights, or expensive workout equipment. This program is based upon the same principles that build the most awesome, powerful, and beautiful bodies of the animal kingdom.

The beauty of Wild Workout® is that it lets you start where you are, at your current level of fitness, and you can use it to reach your fitness goals, whatever they are. If you want huge, bulging muscles like a bull elk, put high tension and muscle resistance into each movement while performing your PowerFlexes. But if your goal is to be toned and sleek like a panther, with healthy muscle definition and shape, ease up on the level of resistance you put into each movement and exercise. You can develop your body the way you want it to be!

Workout Rotation

To get started with Wild Workout®, I recommend that you rotate the sets of exercises that Target the different muscle groups in this fashion:

Week 1: Chest Workout only

Week 2: Chest and Abdominal Workouts

Week 3: Chest, Spine, and Neck Workouts

Week 4: Chest and Back Workouts

Week 5: Chest and Leg Workouts

Week 6: Chest and Shoulder Workouts

Week 7: Chest and Arm Workouts

Week 8: Chest and Speed, Energy, and Endurance Workouts

It's important for you to do the Chest Workout for all eight weeks of this course. This is because the PowerFlexes in the Chest Workout will force you to breathe deeply, which will trigger muscle growth and development throughout your body.

Once you've completed the entire course, now you can become your own best personal trainer! You can now mix and match the exercises that you have learned and target that specific area in your body that you want to enhance, or you can repeat the first cycle again if you wish, or you can replace the Chest Workout with one of the other Workouts, rotating the other Workouts weekly for eight weeks until you've done them all.

Another option is to build your own routine by choosing one exercise from each Workout. Since each of the Workouts in this course contains five PowerFlexes, you have a wide variety to choose from to prevent boredom as you continue to develop your body. Building your own routine allows you to focus on problem areas. For example, if you want to focus on your abdominals, do the whole Abdominal Workout during every session, along with at least one PowerFlex® from each of the other Workouts. Your routine would look like this:

- **Dolphin Flex I**
- **Dolphin Flex II**
- **Shark Flex I**
- **Shark Flex II**
- **Dolphin Flex III**
- **A Chest Exercise**
- **A Spine Exercise**
- **A Neck Exercise**
- **A Back Exercise**
- **A Leg Exercise**
- **A Shoulder Exercise**

- **An Arm Exercise**
- **A Speed, Energy, and Endurance Exercise**

Follow this routine for as long you want, then pick another area to focus on and begin again. The sky's the limit, and it's your body to Build—get creative and use Wild Workout® to your best advantage to build the body you desire!

After you have completed the first 8-weeks open to the back of this book and use Jimmy, John, and Jed's favorite routines to enhance your own body. Also included is specifically designed routines created by these Certified PowerFlex® Personal Trainers to keep you on your lifetime goal of fitness and perform at your top level. They show you how to mix and match this unlimited supply of routines so you never get bored and always moving forward on bettering your body.

Number of Repetitions

Along with instructions for performing each Wild Workout® in this course, there is listed a recommended number of repetitions to do, based on you level of fitness. Level One is for beginners; Level Two is for intermediate, and Level Three is for advanced athletes and those who are well conditioned.

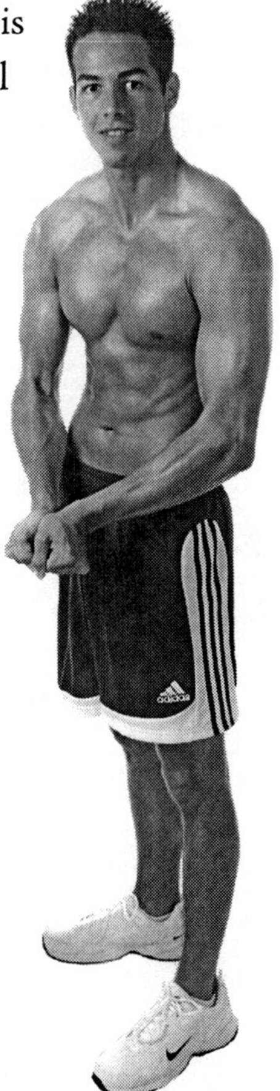

If you can't do the number of repetitions listed for Level One, that's fine—begin your journey where you are. As you do the Wild Workout®, concentrate on the muscles that particular PowerFlex® is designed to work. Use as much resistance as desired for your level of fitness but always remember: "Train, don't Strain!"

It's always good to log your workouts in The PowerFlex® Journal, writing down the PowerFlexes and the number of repetitions you perform so you can track your progress.

Workout Tip: Performing your PowerFlexes in front of a full-length mirror and wear clothing that lets you see your muscles working. Watching yourself while PowerFlexing will help you use proper technique. As you do each PowerFlex®, try to concentrate on the muscles that you are working, this will help you get a much better workout. For example, as you do Gorilla Flex IV (the first bicep PowerFlex® in the Arm Workout), focus your eyes on your biceps as your arm flexes and extends.

Workout Frequency

Some people do two or three Wild Workout® sessions per week. But if you want to see quick improvement, I recommend working out at least five times per week or even six. Wild Workout® can be done anywhere, anytime, and doesn't require special equipment.

You can even PowerFlex® five times per week while watching your favorite half-hour TV show and finish your workout before the show ends! Whether you work out five, three, or two days per week, what matters most is that you're consistent, week in and week out. Stick with it and don't quit! No excuses! Your body will thank you for it a million times over! Your body is like a bank account you only get out of it what you put into it, but with the Wild Workout® you get loads of interest. Now get to it!

HITTING THE BULL'S EYE

The Wild Workout® hits the bull's eye every time with your workouts—That's why you begin to see and feel results faster than you ever imagined possible! This is accomplished by TARGETING the area being worked and using the "Rifle" approach, we zero in on the bulls eye, put that area's muscles in the cross hairs of our scope and targeting specifically that area; we get a fantastic workout. The *Power Arrows* that accompany the illustrations shows you the direction in which to use resistance. If the Power Arrow is pointing up ↑ then resist on the upward motion, if the Power Arrow is Pointing Down ↓ then resist on the downward motion, and if the arrow in both directions resist going both directions. If there are no Power Arrows accompanying the illustration this means your body weight is all the resistance you need while performing this exercise (i.e. The Panther Flex I).

The amazing thing is, that as we see and feel results in that area very quickly we are also working many other muscle groups of our body at the same time, but because we are targeting a certain area and zeroing in on the bulls eye for that area for fast effective unbelievable results, the other muscles being worked are over shadowed but you start noticing results to the entire body.

For example our 1st PowerFlex® the Panther Flex specifically targets the chest muscles, but as your doing the Panther Flex even though it's hitting the bull's eye on the chest region, your also at the same time bringing every muscle into play and giving them a workout your toes, your feet, your calves, your hamstrings, quads, glutes, abs, back, shoulders, neck, arms, hands, and fingers. So as your specifically targeting the chest muscles and hitting the bull's eye seeing amazing results in that area, you're also getting a great workout in the rest of your body. We use the "rifle" approach to zoom in on the target and hit the bull's eye every time!!

Many people wonder why they've been working out for years and yet see no noticeable results, that's because other programs use the "shotgun" approach. Their shooting out a "spread" of BB's trying to hit everything and anything- and they end up hitting nothing. The Wild Workout® TARGETS the section we're working on and yes there is no question the target is a hit a direct Bulls Eye while also working other muscles. The PowerFlex® workout is strategically laid out to bring you the most powerful workout EVER! While working the chest and bringing life giving oxygen to every muscle in the body, you're already preparing your abs for the next workout, while working the abs you're already preparing your neck and spine for the next workouts. While working the neck and spine you're already preparing the back. While working the back you're already preparing the legs, while working the legs you're already preparing the shoulders. While working the shoulders you're already preparing the arms, and when you get to the speed energy and endurance workout every muscle group that you've been through gets a phenomenal workout tying everything together. Plus when you move from one section to another, the section you're moving on from still comes into play as you begin your next workout so you never lose what you've just accomplished. It's AWESOME!!!

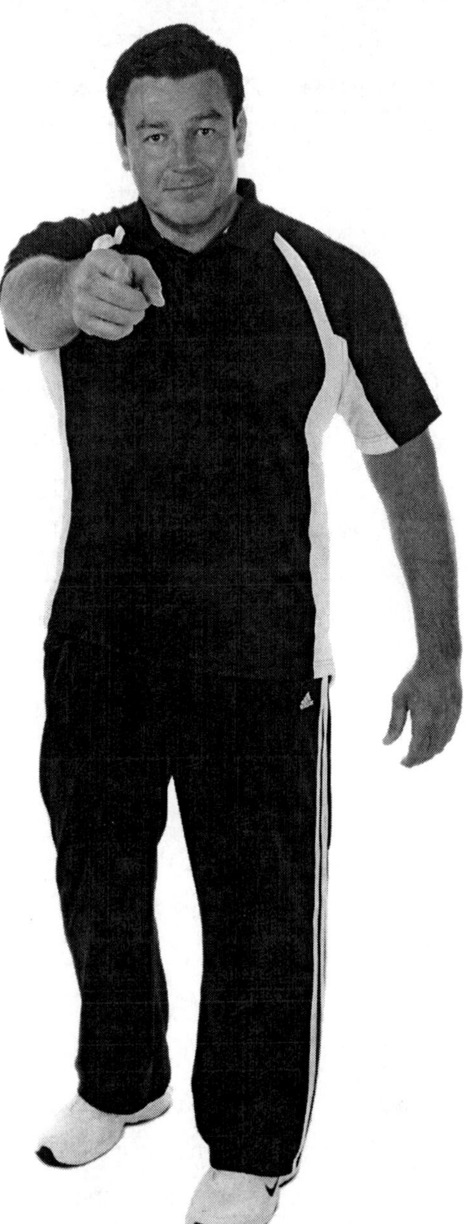

TAKE BACK YOUR BODY

My friend, you can have the BODY YOU DESIRE! It is not a myth, a fairytale, or a fable. Nobody has cornered the market on having a great body—nobody! Having a superb body is not just for movie stars, athletes, the rich, the famous, and everybody but you. You might be saying, "Oh, I've tried to get myself in shape before, but it never worked." Listen, my friend, Thomas Edison went through over 1,000 filaments trying to find one that would work in a light bulb, and then he finally found THE ONE that worked, produced results, and was the REAL DEAL!

You might have tried 1,000 other workout programs, but now you have found THE ONE that works, produces results, and is the REAL DEAL! The results you begin to very quickly achieve will be enough to keep you motivated to keep on going. Here's the truth: your body will respond *very quickly*. If all you get out of this program is to go for a brisk mile walk a day, throw out your soda, and drink at least eight glasses of PURE natural water, you will be amazed at the transformation these simple steps alone will bring you! And this program, my friend, gives you *oh so much more!* Use Wild Workout® to its full advantage and TAKE BACK YOUR BODY. When you begin to see and feel the fantastic results, when you begin to hear the compliments and notice people taking second glances at you, that alone will steer you away from bad food and drink choices and keep you going in the right direction. It's awesome! Now TAKE BACK YOUR BODY.

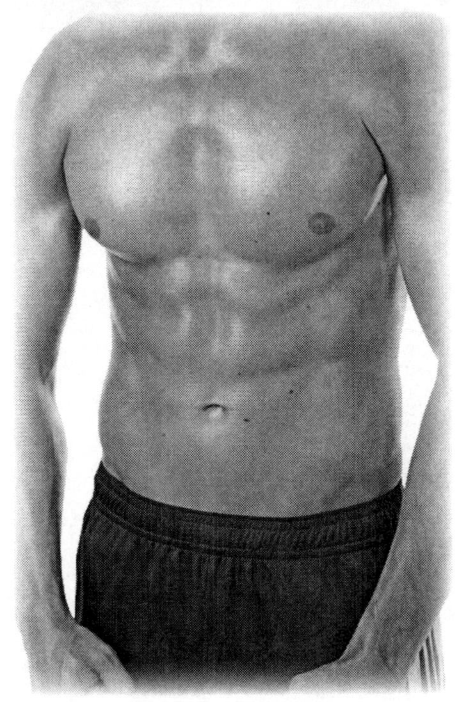

4 SECRETS OF HEALTH

There are four secrets to health that are so simple, yet so effective—constantly refer to them, practice them, and make them part of your lifestyle, and you will be amazed at how easy it is to be and remain healthy! Being healthy is not found in trying out fad diets and chasing fancy and expensive trends. It is making solid healthy decisions on a consistent basis. Being healthy is a lifestyle, and when these four secrets become a part of your regular decisions, they will make all the difference in the world. Take them seriously and make them a part of your life starting today.

SECRET #1—EXERCISE

The human body was created to last a long time. It's one of the only things in the universe that gets BETTER the more you use it! Experts agree that exercise will help:

- **Keep your weight under control**
- **Reduce your risk of heart disease, diabetes, and high blood pressure**
- **Improve your blood cholesterol levels**
- **Prevent bone loss**
- **Boost your energy levels**
- **Manage tension**
- **Improve self-image**
- **Control anxiety**
- **Control depression**

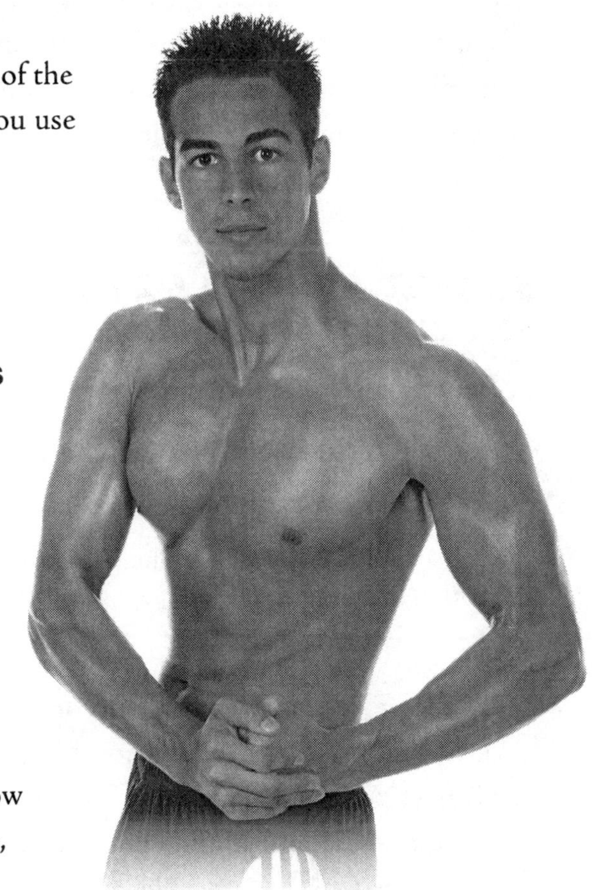

Exercise on a regular basis. The only things that don't move are rocks and the dead! Exercise regularly. You now have PowerFlex®, which can be done anywhere at anytime, so NO EXCUSES!

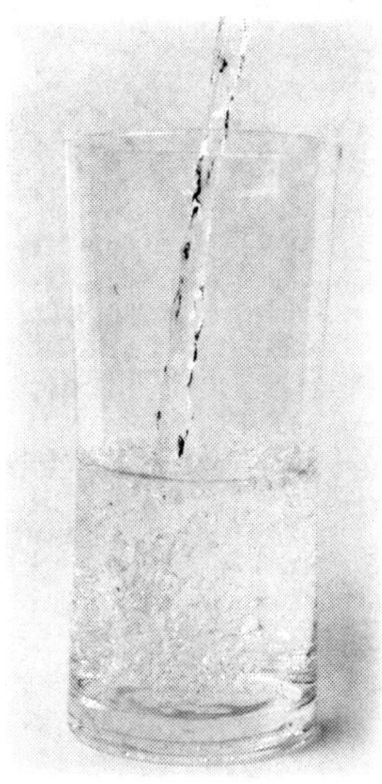

SECRET #2—DRINK ENOUGH PURE WATER EVERY DAY

Experts agree that our bodies require a minimum of at least eight glasses of pure water a day. If you are very active and involved in strenuous exercise, you should drink much more than that. After all, seventy percent of your body is made up of water—not protein, not carbs, not meat, or anything else. PURE WATER is liquid life. Through daily sweating, breathing, carrying oxygen to muscles, helping to digest food, flushing waste products from the body, lubricating joints, and so much more, so much of our water is lost daily. Even if you are a couch potato, your water level must be replenished—eight glasses a day minimum.

The next time you are at the store, and your hand is reaching for a soda, say, "No. I will grab a water drink instead." It is now available everywhere in a variety of forms—spring, artesian, natural, bottled at source, carbonated, flavored with pure fruit juices, in a bottle, in a can, by the gallon, six pack, case—at the office, delivered to your home in five-gallon jugs. It's everywhere. So there is no excuse to not pass on the soda and sugar drinks and drink eight glasses of pure water a day. It's more important than your diet. Because seventy percent of you is water, give yourself a break and drink some!

SECRET #3—STAY AWAY FROM WHITE BREAD, WHITE SUGAR, AND WHITE FLOUR

Experts agree that there are many healthier choices than "white" foods:

White bread—rather, choose whole wheat, whole grain, rye, pumpernickel, multigrain, etc.

White sugar—rather, choose honey, brown sugar, unprocessed cane sugar, etc.

White flour—rather, choose whole wheat noodles, spinach noodles, brown rice, etc.

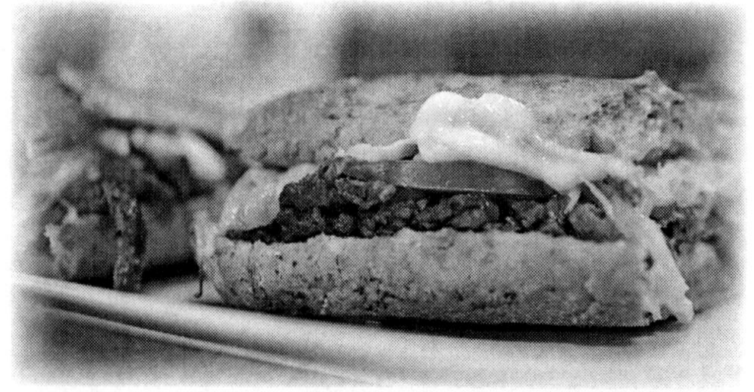

It's the processing, bleaching, etc. of the white products that make them an unwise choice. Many people have pounds and pounds of waste stuck in their intestines because of their poor diet of these types of foods—plus they are clogged!

The healthy choices are not only good for you and add nutrients to your body, but they also help to keep you clean inside and properly cleansed within. The healthy choices are everywhere and conveniently available from supermarkets to restaurants. So no excuses—choose healthy.

Ask for a whole wheat bun for your burger. Yes, the fast food places will give you one. You only have to ask. Ask for whole wheat noodles with your pasta. Ask for spinach noodles, ask for honey, ask for a whole wheat crust in your pizza. Get your sandwich on multigrain bread. You have not because you ask not! No excuses!

SECRET #4—EAT BAKED, NOT FRIED

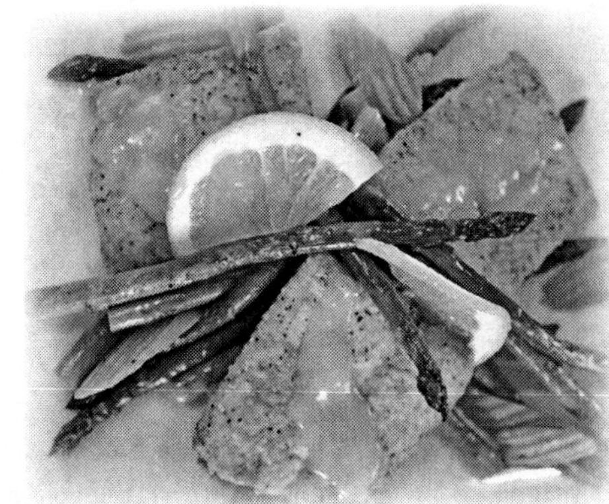

Experts agree that the frying of foods is what soaks everything full of grease, fat, and lard! Go for a baked potato, not French fries. Go for baked chips, not fried. Go for baked, grilled, broiled, or flame-broiled lean meat, fish, turkey, steak, or chicken—anything but fried and deep fried.

Use virgin olive oil instead of lard. It's your choice. Make it—no excuses! Plus you can snack all you want, if you snack on the right healthy foods.

Here's a list to help you:

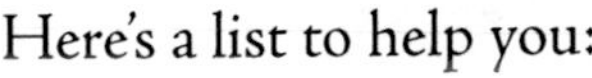

FRUITS

Apples
Plums
Coconut
Tangerines
Strawberries
Melons
Grapes
Oranges
Kiwi
Nectarines
Berries
Raspberries
Grapefruit
Bananas

VEGETABLES

Cauliflower
Carrots
Broccoli
Green peppers

Lettuce
Cucumbers
Peas
Beets
Celery
Cabbage
Green beans
Radishes

RAW NUTS and SEEDS

Sunflower seeds
Almonds
Cashews
Walnuts
Hazel nuts
Brazilian nuts
Hickory nuts
Peanuts in the shell

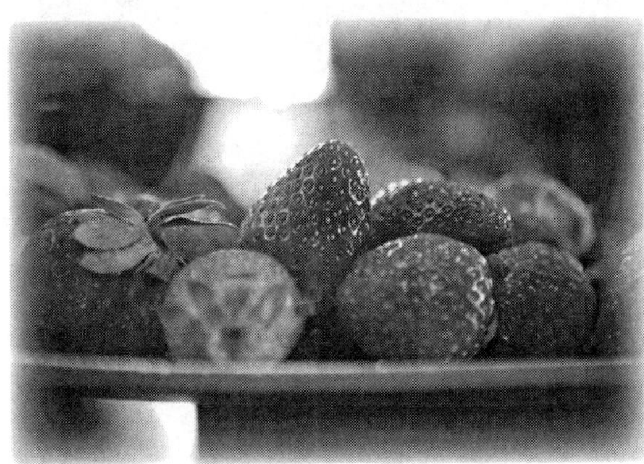

Just be careful you are not loading up your snack choices with fattening sauces and dips and that the seeds and nuts are not coated with salt or candied. Every grocery store now has a wide selection of these healthy snacks, so go load up on them. Leave your excuses behind!

3 MOTIVATION TIPS THAT WORK

My friend, be prepared to face the fact that there will be days when you flat out won't want to exercise. You just won't feel like it. Here are three fantastic tips that will overcome that deflated feeling and get you to exercise anyway, and you will be so glad you did. These work, so use them!

MOTIVATION TIP #1

Have a set of exercise clothes that are for the exclusive purpose of wearing when you exercise and for nothing else—not for knocking around the house, not for going out in public. The only purpose of these clothes is for exercise. I have many sets of shorts, T-shirts, and tank tops that I only wear when exercising. Why? What you wear determines how you act.

When wearing a tuxedo, you don't feel much like playing tackle football. When wearing your favorite ripped jeans and T-shirt with your comfortable tennis shoes, you don't feel much like standing around in church. What you wear determines your mind-set, and when you are having one of those days when you're looking for an excuse to not exercise, go put your exercise clothes on. Your mind-set will begin to change.

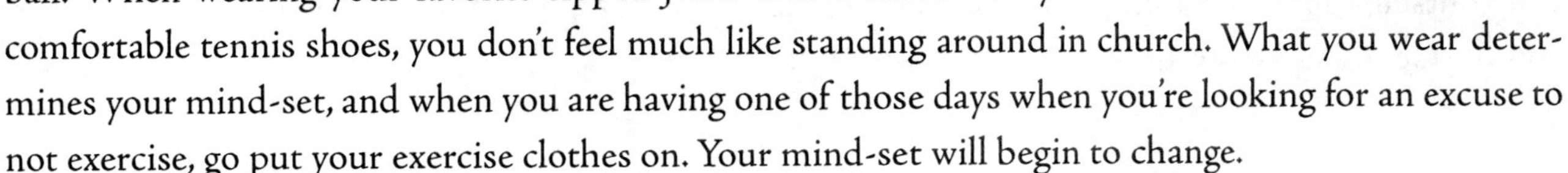

MOTIVATION TIP #2

Turn on your favorite music and crank it up! When you think you have it loud, give it another boost even louder. Push the volume to the verge of being obnoxious. Your favorite music blasting will begin to overcome your deflated feeling, your mood will shift gears, and your attitude will change. Even little babies can't keep still when they hear good music—they begin to smile, bounce up and down, and move to the beat. Use that power of music for yourself, and your motivation will greatly surprise you!

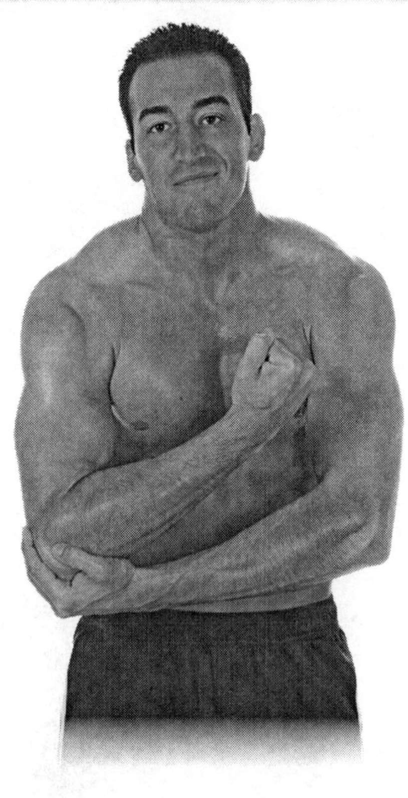

MOTIVATION TIP #3

The human body is so advanced you can't begin to comprehend how great it is. Your body is already programmed to fill in the gaps. Whenever you watched a movie, you might have thought you saw all the action and movement, but you actually only saw still pictures, and your mind filled in the gap between them to make them appear in full action. That's why subliminal messages were outlawed from movies, because even though they were too fast for a person's eye to see, people's minds saw them, and they were affected.

Theaters used to flash soda or popcorn ads during movies, and people would get thirsty or want popcorn. Even though their eyes didn't see them, their minds picked up on the images. Use this advanced knowledge to your advantage. When you don't feel like exercising, tell yourself, "Well, I'll get my exercise clothes on, crank up my music, and I'll exercise. But I'm going to take it slow. I'm not going to break any records. I'm not going to push myself today. I'll take it easy and just get them done."

When you start to do your workouts during these times, you'll find you have some of your very best workouts. You get started, take the pressure off by telling yourself you are just going to take it easy, and your body takes over and fills in the gaps. When you're done, you'll smile and say, "Wow! That was an awesome workout. I'm glad I did it!" Put on your exercise clothes. Crank up the music. Tell yourself you're not going to break any records today. These helpful hints will get you over the hump! Use them! No excuses!

OUR MISSION

"Wild Workout® is dedicated to empowering each person to build the body they desire—whether that body is massively muscled like a bull elk, or lean, sculpted, and toned like a panther. Wild Workout® is dedicated to empowering people to build strength, health, and fitness naturally by using their body's own energies and abilities—as the beautiful creatures of the animal kingdom do."

Welcome to the Wild Workout® I commend you for having the courage to take the step that your body will reward you for an entire lifetime. It is always a great pleasure to know there are people such as you, who take control of their lives and health and go forward with confidence. Wild Workout® is the most revolutionary and powerful way to exercise for fast, powerful, eye-popping results. Yet the principle behind Wild Workout® is so simple. It is so simple and powerful, in fact, that mankind has overlooked it for centuries.

The most powerful, graceful, awe-inspiring, perfectly sculpted specimens of strength and beauty—that capture the stares of on looking eyes —is not that of the human specimen, but the grace and beauty and strength found in the animal kingdom. From the awesome strength, grace, and beauty of the Lion whom the "Good Book" calls the strongest of beasts, to the mesmerizing muscles and agility of the majestic Elk who roam the top of mountains as if its child's play though they weigh-in at over 1,000 pounds. Yet when you consider the pillars of strength, the flexibility, the incredible speed, the ripped muscles, and the beauty of creatures among the animal kingdom, you'll notice there is no workout gym, no special equipment, no weights, no bars, no bands, no machines or dumbbells. It is all attained by using their own bodies' energies and abilities to bend, twist, push, pull, flex, and move. It is this same principle that Wild Workout® is built upon, and make no mistake, it works—no ifs ands or buts. It's not up for questions or debate. The animals have already proven the point a million times, and it worked for me.

Based upon my physique alone, I was offered a full scholarship by the chancellor of a major East Coast college that turns out many professional football players. My chest muscles and upper body strength and overall look was gained through the Wild Workout® program, and the college chancellor was impressed. He wanted me on a plane within two days if I would be the fullback of their team.

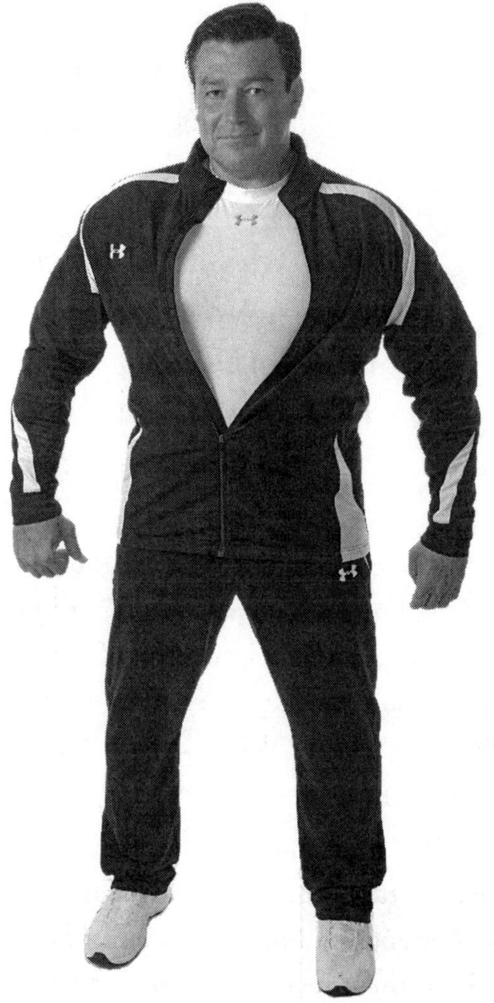

I turned down the gracious offer, to pursue my father's business, and I've turned down other offers since then. I've also coached and quarterbacked my own city league team to five championships and raised it to be one of the most feared and respected teams in the league. Because of Wild Workout® and the energy and glow and respectability it has given me as a person, I've grown accustomed to the notices, advances, and opportunities that come my way that others dream about, not only myself but now also my family who follow the same program and are the heart of this book.

This program is not bound by any type of barriers not even generation barriers as you see my family is now reaching greater heights of accomplishments than I did as you will see throughout the book. Wherever we are, we are constantly approached and have doors opened for us by people who mistake us for professional athletes, Olympic weightlifters, bodybuilders, professional wrestlers, actors, or models. Our physiques gets their attention, and they think that we must be someone special.

Countless people have approached us and asked how many hours we spend in the gym a day, how much we bench press, and how we attained this level of physical fitness. Knowing that a proud arrogant braggart is the most unattractive person in the world, I usually respond to their inquiries by saying,"I'm on the George Foreman workout program— McDonalds for breakfast and Burger King for lunch." Seriously, though, after you've sculpted your muscles, please feel free to tell your admirers that it's due to Wild Workout®. Now let's get to it!

POWERFLEX Chest

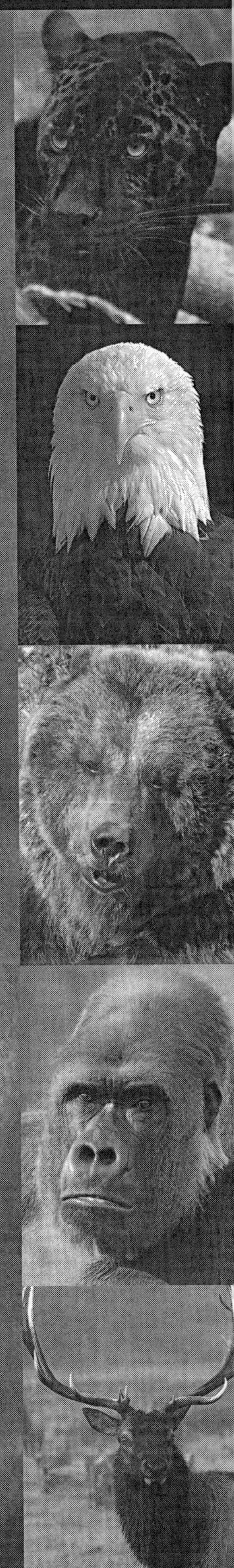

CHEST WORKOUT

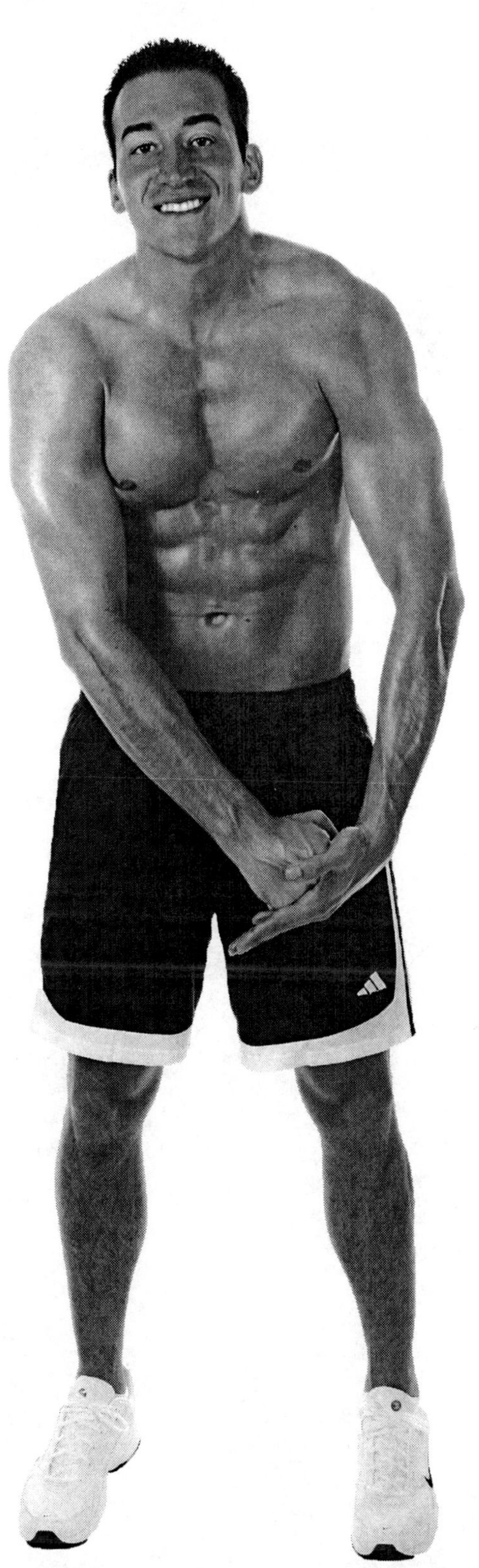

The Wild Workout® program for building a huge, powerful, massive chest, without special equipment or steroids, is based on the principle of five of the most powerful animals that possess massive chest strength—the panther, eagle, bear, gorilla, and elk. All you need are 5 simple PowerFlexes, 20 minutes per day, and your own best effort!

#1—PANTHER FLEX I

You'll notice when a panther or any member of the cat family gets ready to strike their prey, they crouch and flex their massive chest muscles that give them such extraordinary leaping ability as they spring upon their mark. The Panther Flex stimulates that flex for the chest. We've all done push-ups from time to time—well now get ready to take the humble push-up to the next level.

To do the Panther Flex, do push-ups between two chairs (or any sturdy objects of equal height). Set your chairs just a little wider than shoulder-width apart and let your body sink a little lower than the chairs as you go down. It's this extra flex that feeds and nourishes and works your chest muscles with staggering results. Don't be fooled, this PowerFlex® will give you what you're looking for. It's for real.

LEVEL THREE: 100 repetitions
LEVEL TWO: 40 repetitions
LEVEL ONE: 20 repetitions

Sometimes I do 100 repetitions all at once, and other times I break up those repetitions into sets, resting a bit between each set (70 + 30, or 50 + 50, or 30 + 40 + 30, etc.). Feel free to break up your repetitions into sets, too. Experiment to see what works for you and don't do more than you're comfortable with. What matters most is that you do your Wild Workout® consistently—day after day, week after week, month after month. You won't have long to wait, though, before your consistency and patience start to reap their rewards.

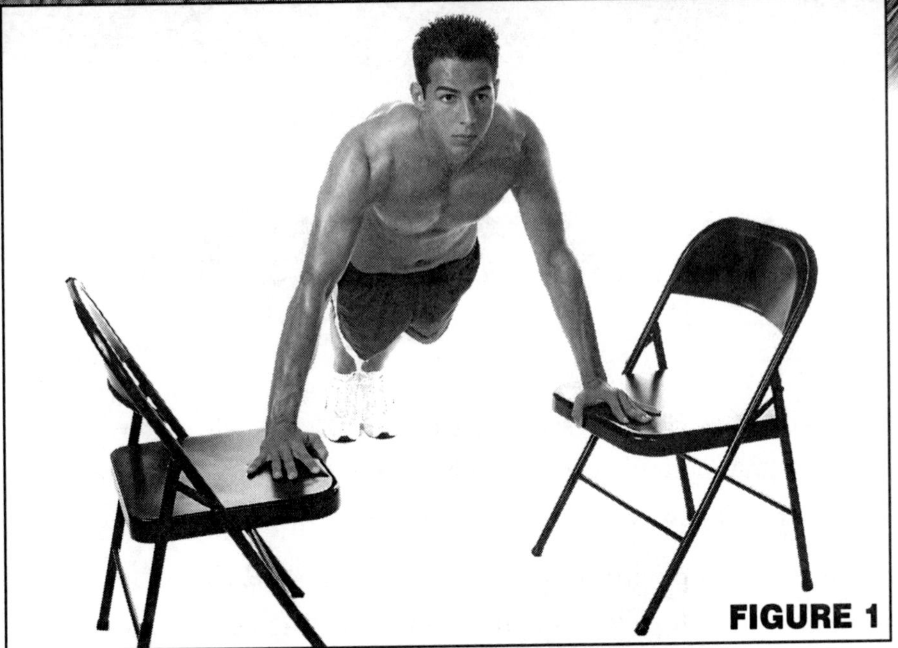
FIGURE 1

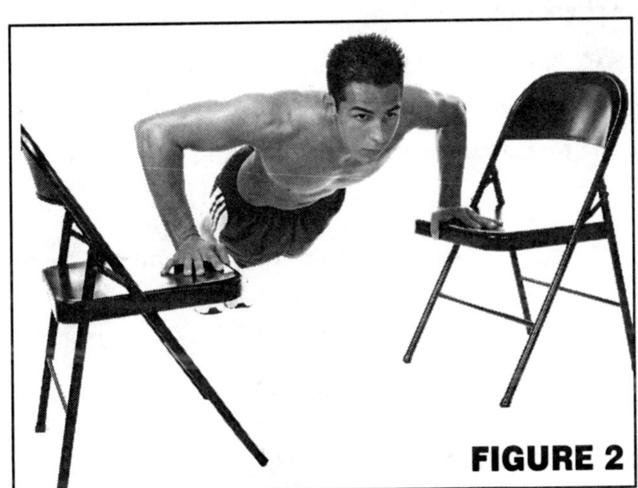
FIGURE 2

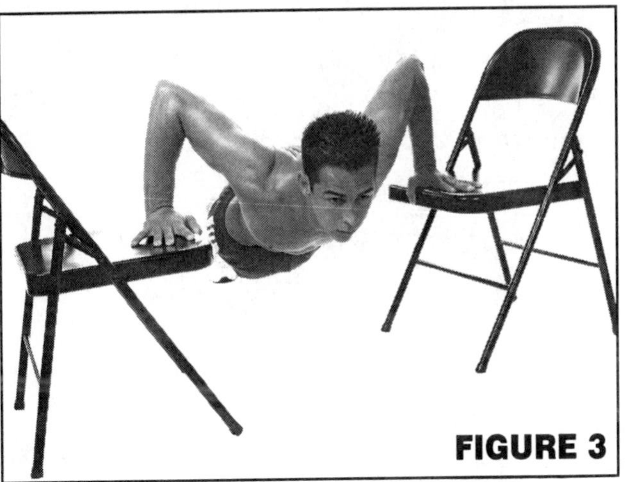
FIGURE 3

Advanced

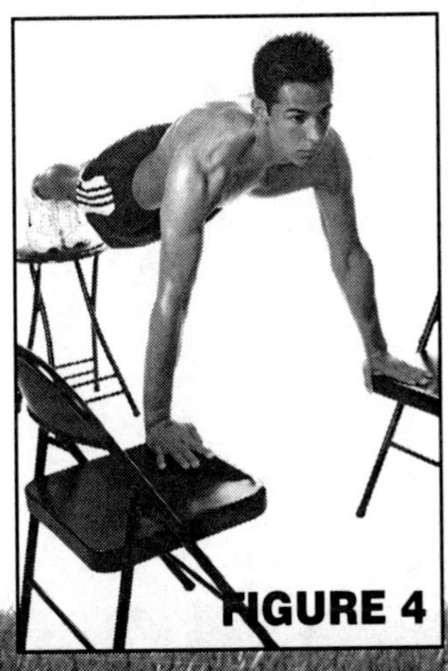
FIGURE 4

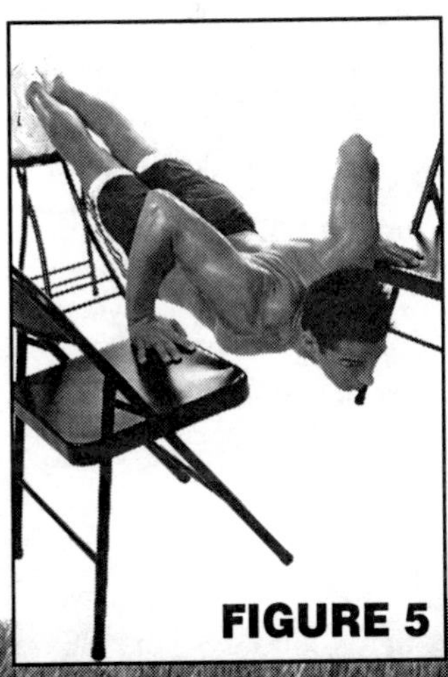
FIGURE 5

Modified

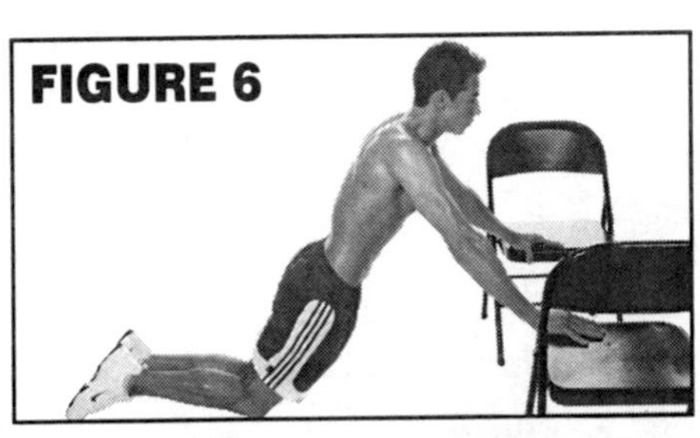
FIGURE 6

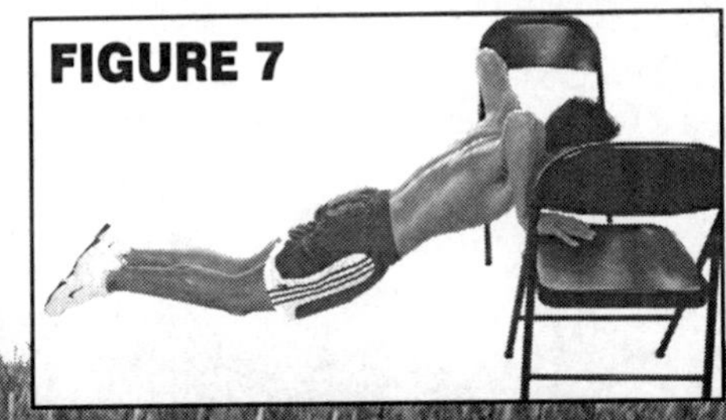
FIGURE 7

#2—EAGLE FLEX I

It's no wonder that the eagle is the symbol of the greatest country on earth. Its massive chest strength carries it to great heights—even above mountaintops. It accomplishes this by flexing its chest muscles over and over and over again as its massive wings go up and down stimulating the chest.

To perform the Eagle Flex, stand straight up with your feet shoulder-width apart and your arms straight down at your sides. With fingers extending with an open hand, slowly raise your arms, keeping them straight as an eagle's wing, while flexing your chest muscles. Reach and extend farther as you raise your arms and extend them as wings. Extend them until your hands are just a little higher than your head, then bring your arms down slightly in front of you, now flexing your chest muscles on the way down, until your hands cross in front of you. Breathe in as you go up—fill your lungs—and exhale as you come down.

Reverse the movement and repeat. This exercise develops the chest muscles quickly, and the deep breathing it involves will stimulate muscle growth throughout your body.

LEVEL THREE: 60 repetitions
LEVEL TWO: 30 repetitions
LEVEL ONE: 15 repetitions

REMEMBER: If your goal is to develop a massive, imposing physique, you'll need to use more resistance while doing your PowerFlexes than someone whose goal is to develop more of a lean, and toned physique.

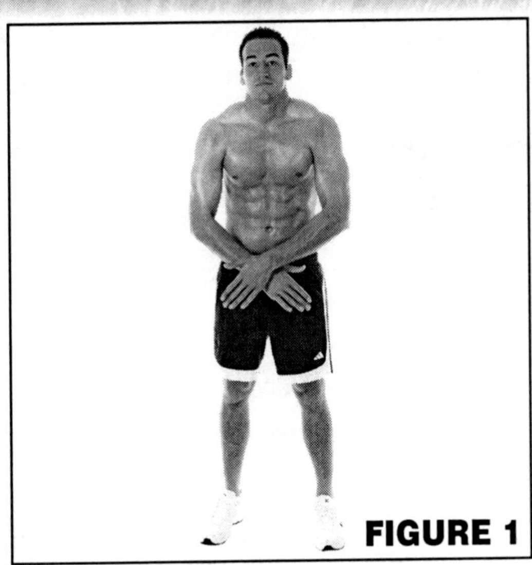
FIGURE 1

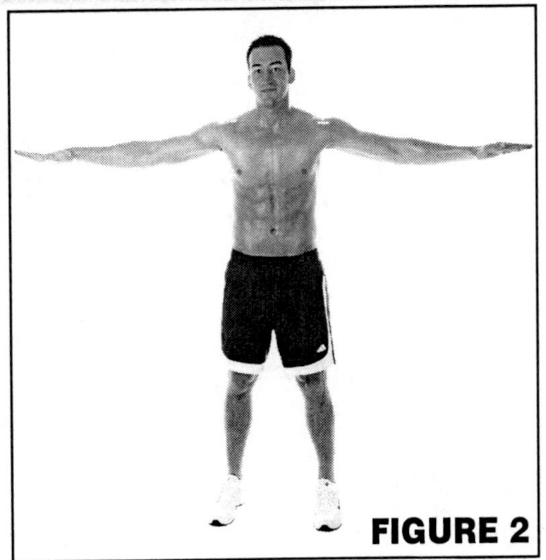
FIGURE 2

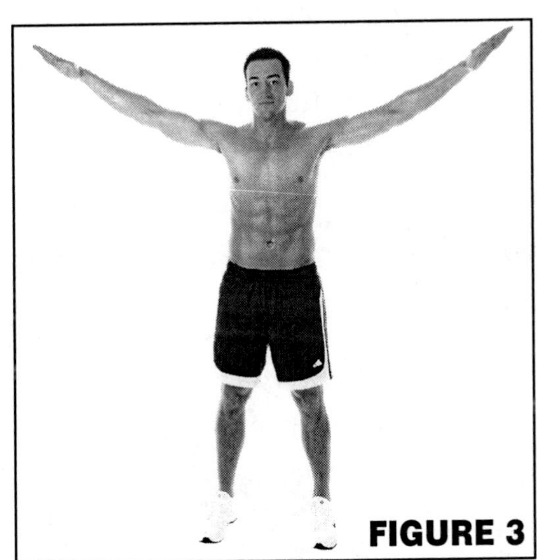
FIGURE 3

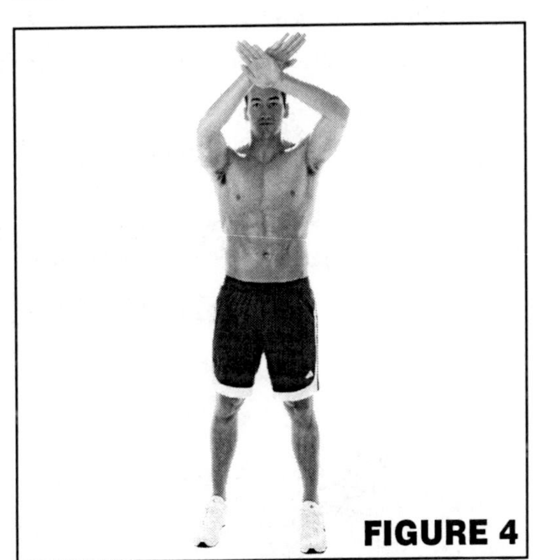
FIGURE 4

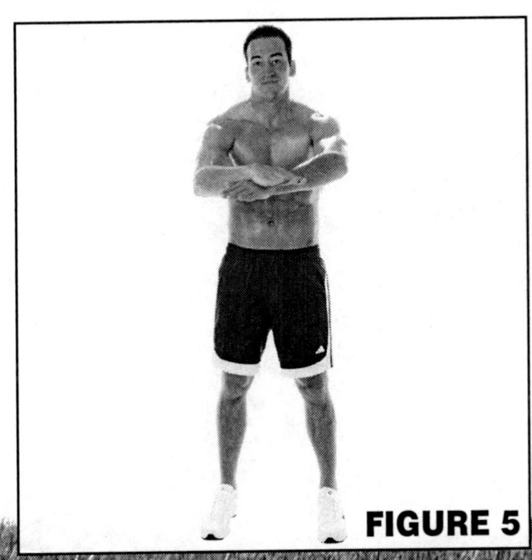
FIGURE 5

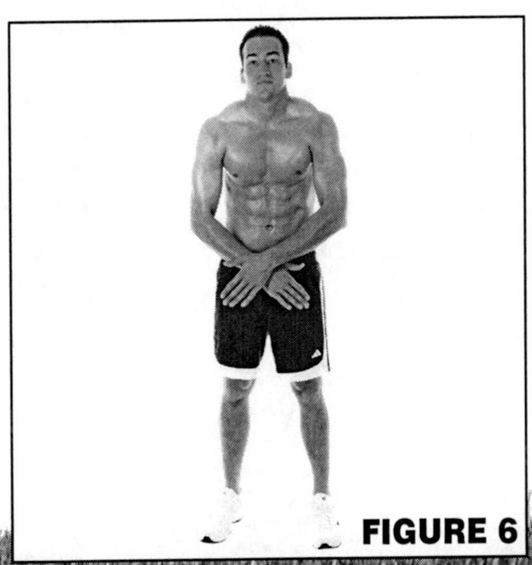
FIGURE 6

#3—BEAR FLEX I

There's only one way to describe the bone crushing power of something that has the strength to take your breath away with a squeeze it's called the bear hug. This massive barrel-chested creature is admired and feared around the world for its loveableness and awesome ability to crush anything in the massive hug of its chests.

The Bear Flex I simulates a bear hug. Stand with your hands in front of you, a little lower than your waist. With one hand turned up and the other turned down, grip and interlock your fingers in a cupped position. With your fingers locked and pulling apart, slowly lift your hands while keeping them close to your body until your hands are over your head, flexing your chest muscles as you do it. Keep the tension on, pulling apart with fingers interlocked. Then slowly move back down to the starting position.

LEVEL THREE: 40 repetitions
LEVEL TWO: 25 repetitions
LEVEL ONE: 10 repetitions

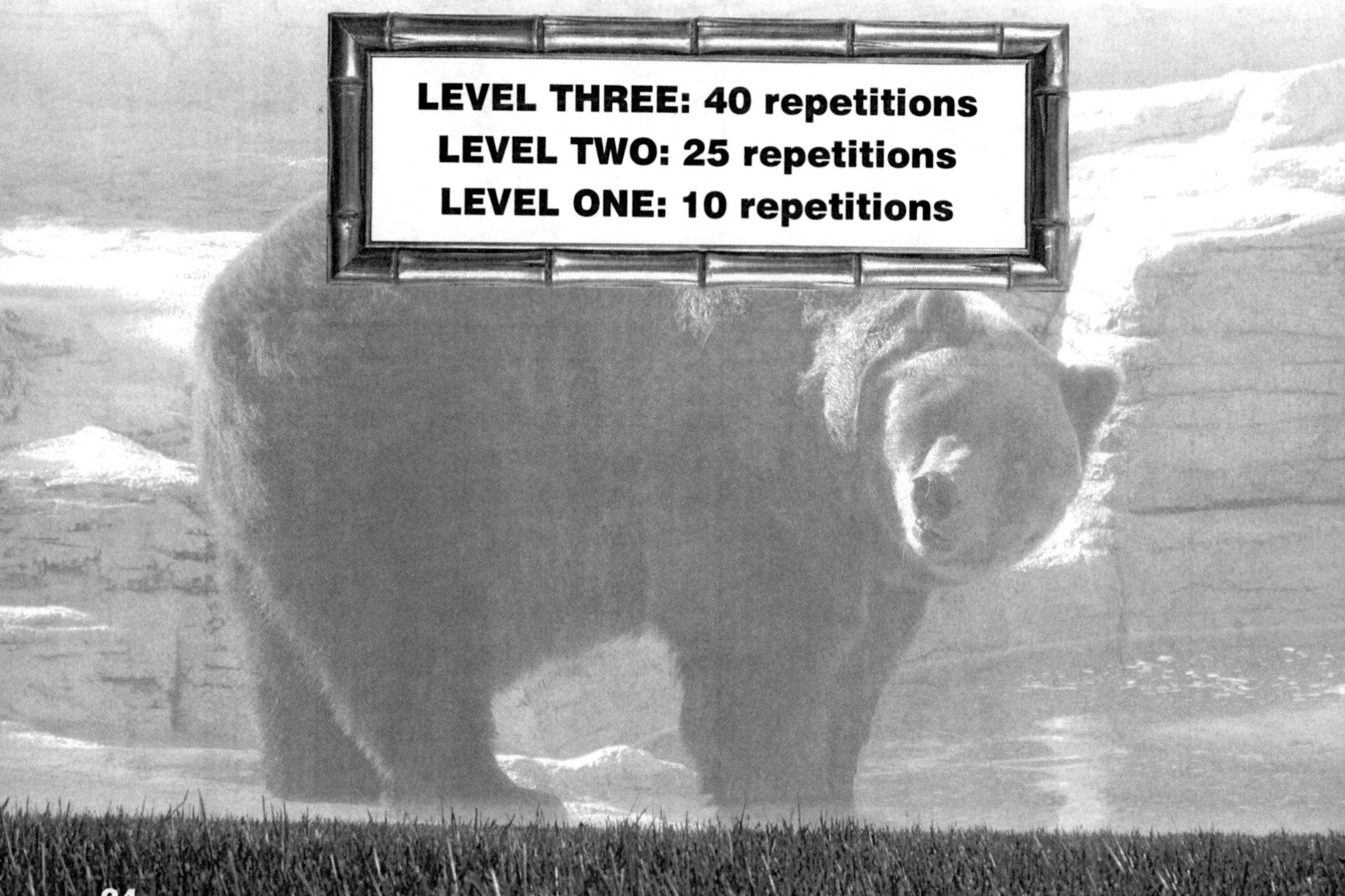

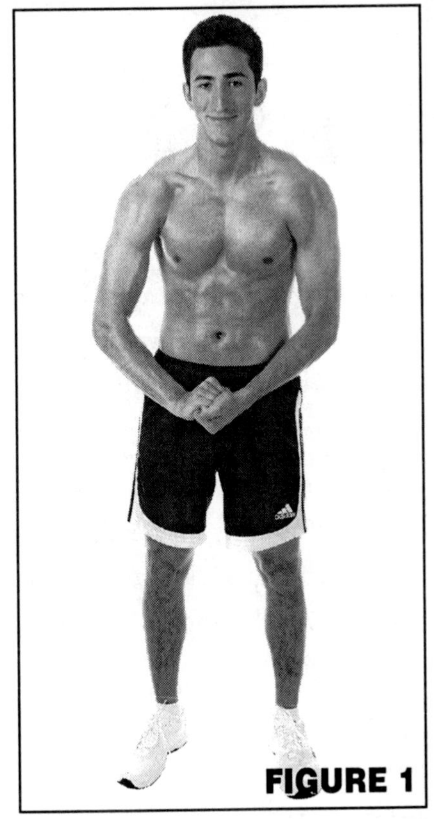
FIGURE 1

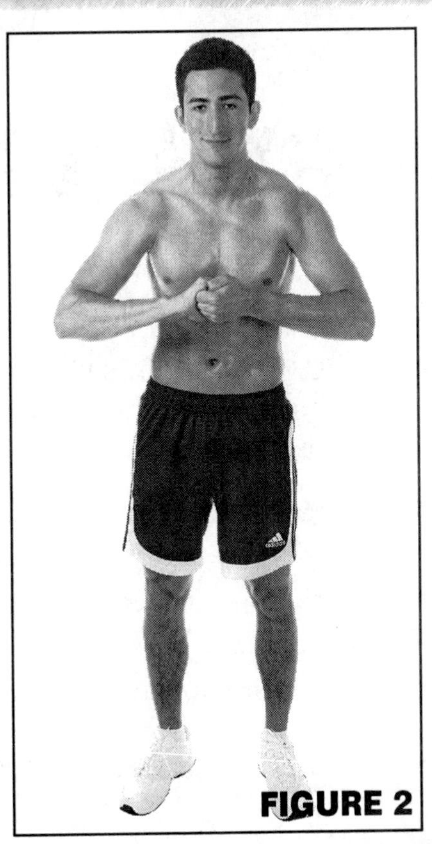
FIGURE 2

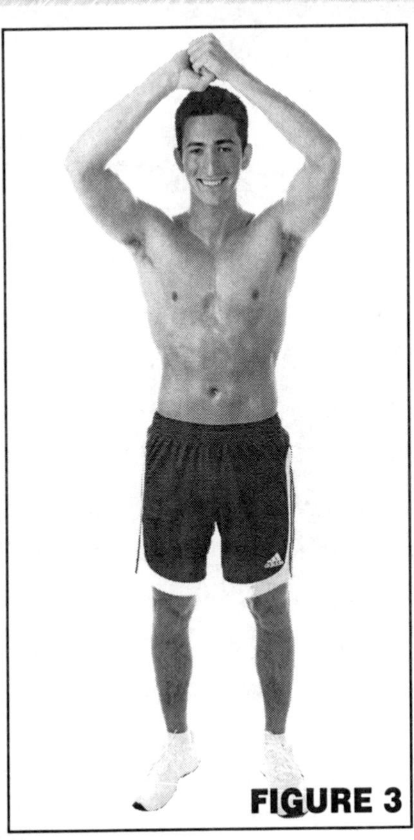
FIGURE 3

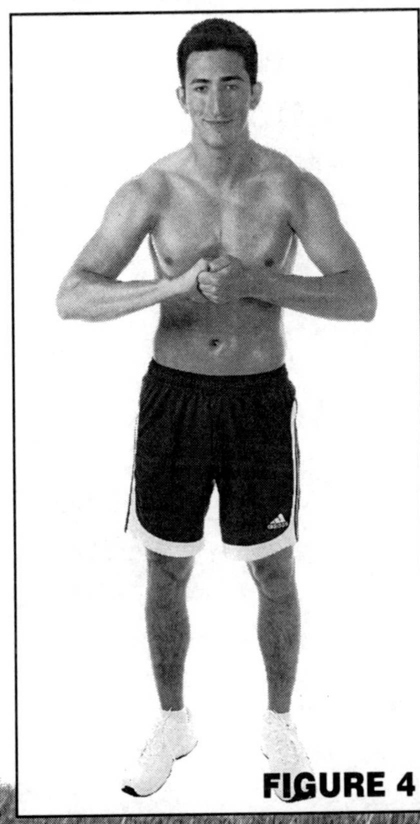
FIGURE 4

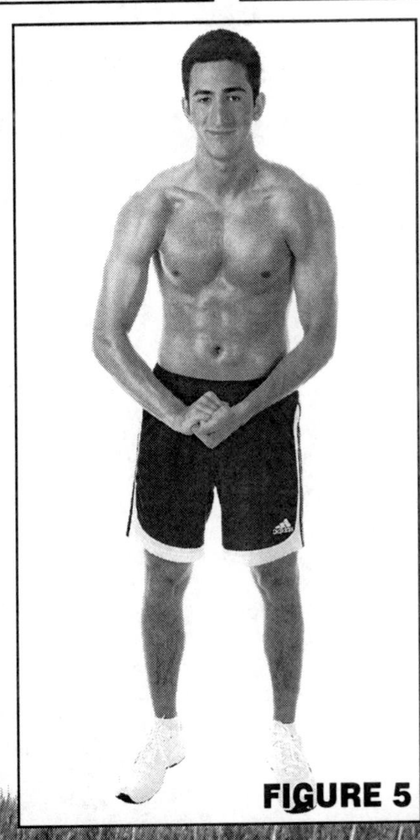
FIGURE 5

#4—GORILLA FLEX I

The massive gorilla pounds proudly on his immense chest to display his superiority. Considering their size, gorillas display mind-boggling strength and agility through their swinging, climbing, and pulling itself up vines and branches. Fortunately, you don't need vines, branches, or special equipment to simulate this movement, thanks to the Gorilla Flex I.

Imagine there's a climbing rope hanging in front of you. Standing with your feet shoulder width apart, grab that imaginary rope, clinch it in your fists tightly in front of you just above your head. Then flex your chest muscles as you slowly pull that rope down resisting your top hand against your bottom hand as you pull down in front of you. Flex, pull, and grip with each hand, alternately, until both hands are a bit lower than your waist. Raise your hands above your head again and repeat.

LEVEL THREE: 40 repetitions
LEVEL TWO: 20 repetitions
LEVEL ONE: 10 repetitions

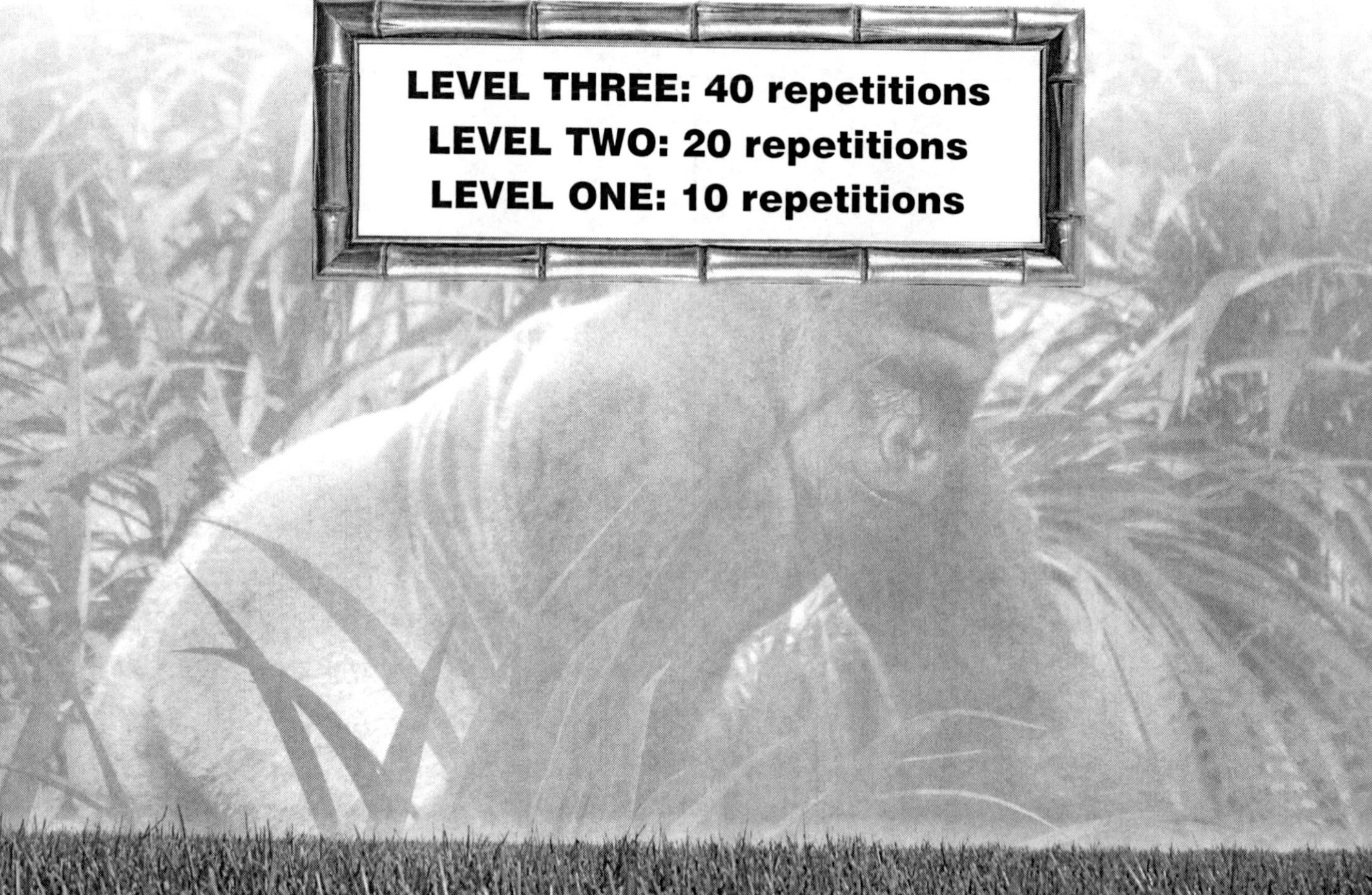

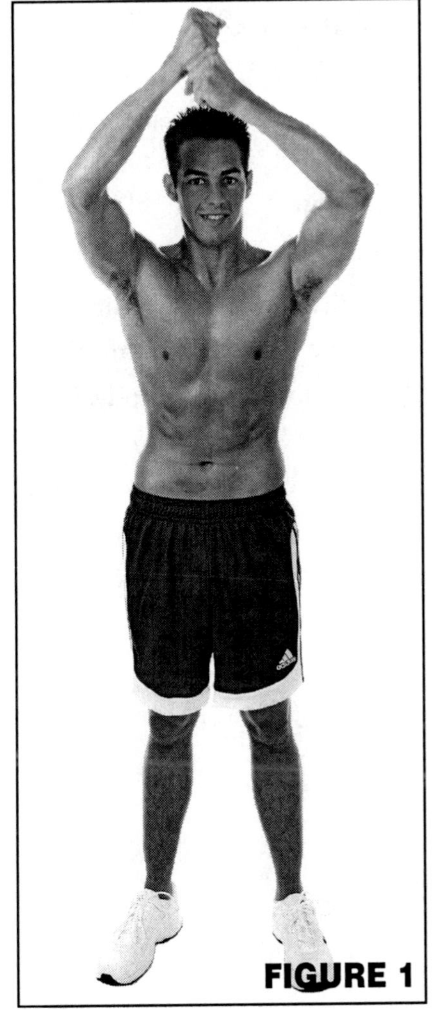
FIGURE 1

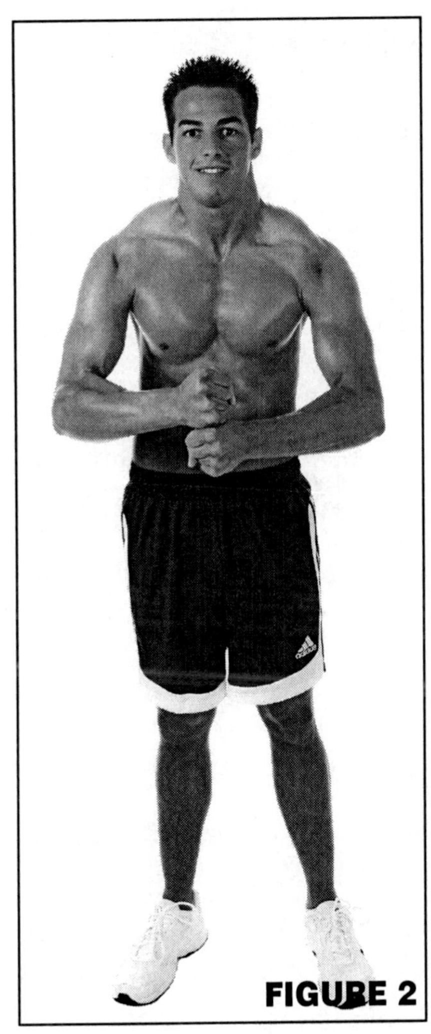
FIGURE 2

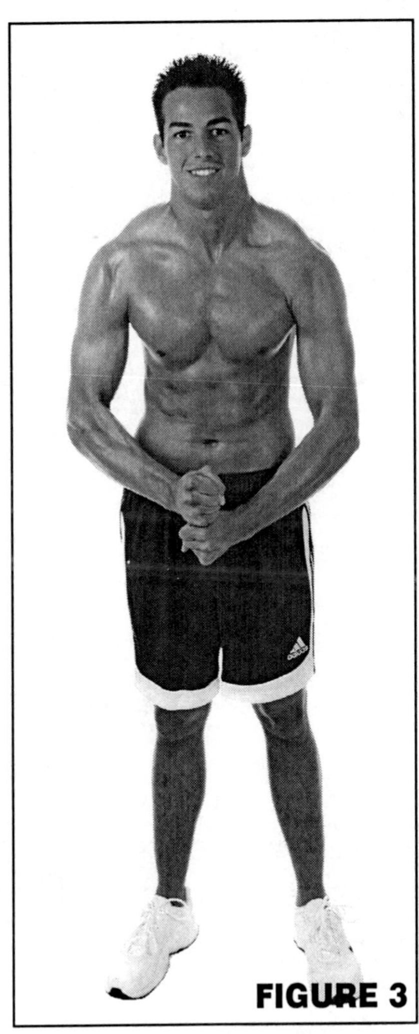
FIGURE 3

#5—BULL ELK FLEX I

One glimpse of a bull elk in the wild is enough to make the strongest heart feel faint! It's no wonder it's called and described with words like; majestic, royal, elusive, it is absolutely awesome! Its indescribably massive chest gives it the ability to climb mountaintops at over 10,000 feet with ease.

The Bull Elk Flex I brings into play the working of the elk's chest as he flexes his chest against the resistance of climbing the mountain. Make a fist with one hand and place the fist in the palm of the other hand, with your knuckles on the palm and the inside of the fisted hand close to your body. Keep your upper arms straight at your sides, slightly ahead of you, bending only at the elbows. Start with the palm of the hand about chest high, then push down on that palm with your fist, resisting the fist with the palm and flexing your chest muscles, just as a bull elk goes up a mountainside. Slowly allow the fist to overcome the palm, forcing the arm down slowly until it is a little lower than your waist. Now do the same exercise on the other side, reversing the position of your hands.

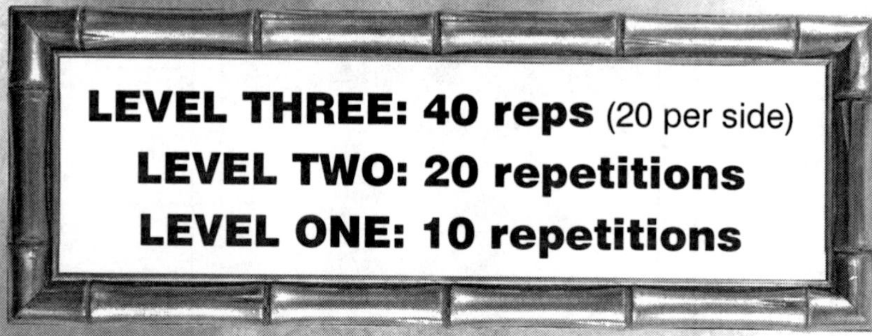

LEVEL THREE: 40 reps (20 per side)
LEVEL TWO: 20 repetitions
LEVEL ONE: 10 repetitions

Performing these five PowerFlexes with consistency, determination, and patience will earn you the chest development you desire—all without steroids, special equipment, or even a gym membership. It won't be long before you see the fruit of your labors. Please feel free to discuss on the Wild Workout® Forum, write, or email me and let me know how you're progressing. I want to rejoice in your progress with you!

However far along you are with Wild Workout®, I want to commend you again for your determination to improve your fitness, appearance, and health—to "walk the walk," not just "talk the talk"!

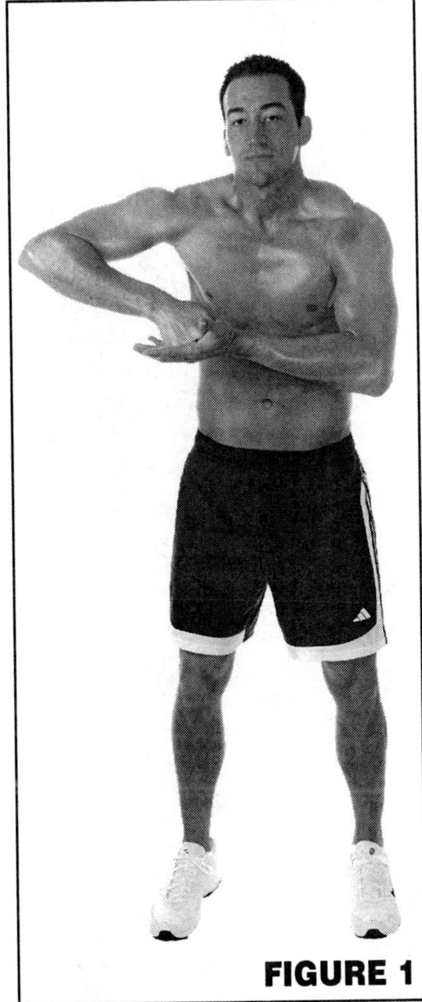
FIGURE 1

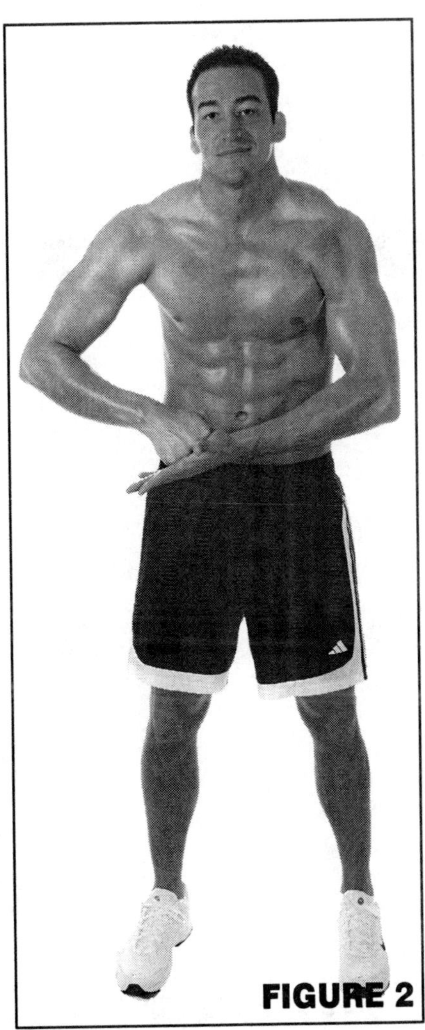
FIGURE 2

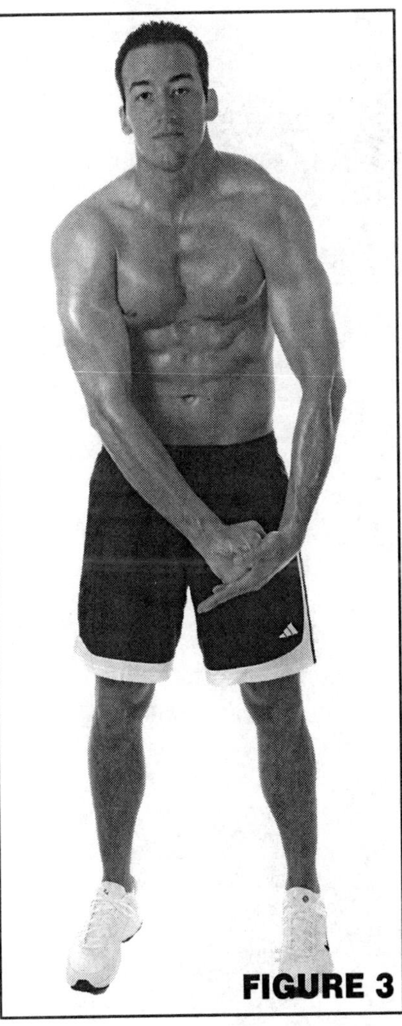
FIGURE 3

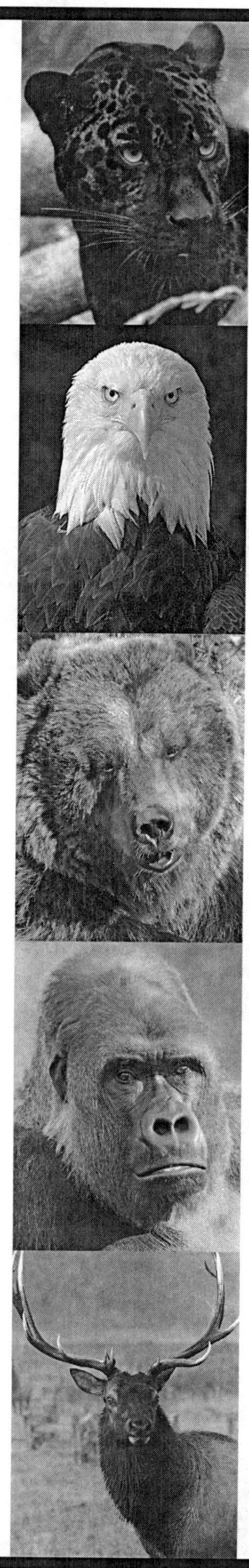

Chest Exercises

PANTHER FLEX I

EAGLE FLEX I

BEAR FLEX I

GORILLA FLEX I

ELK FLEX I

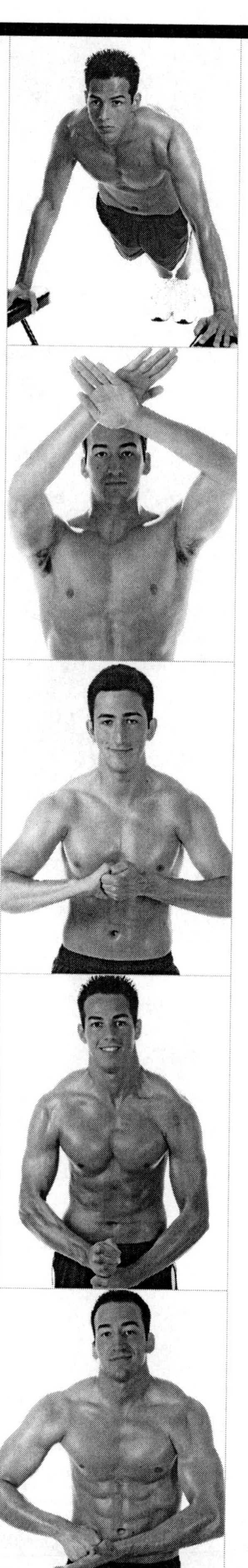

POWERFLEX
Abdominals

ABDOMINALS WORKOUT

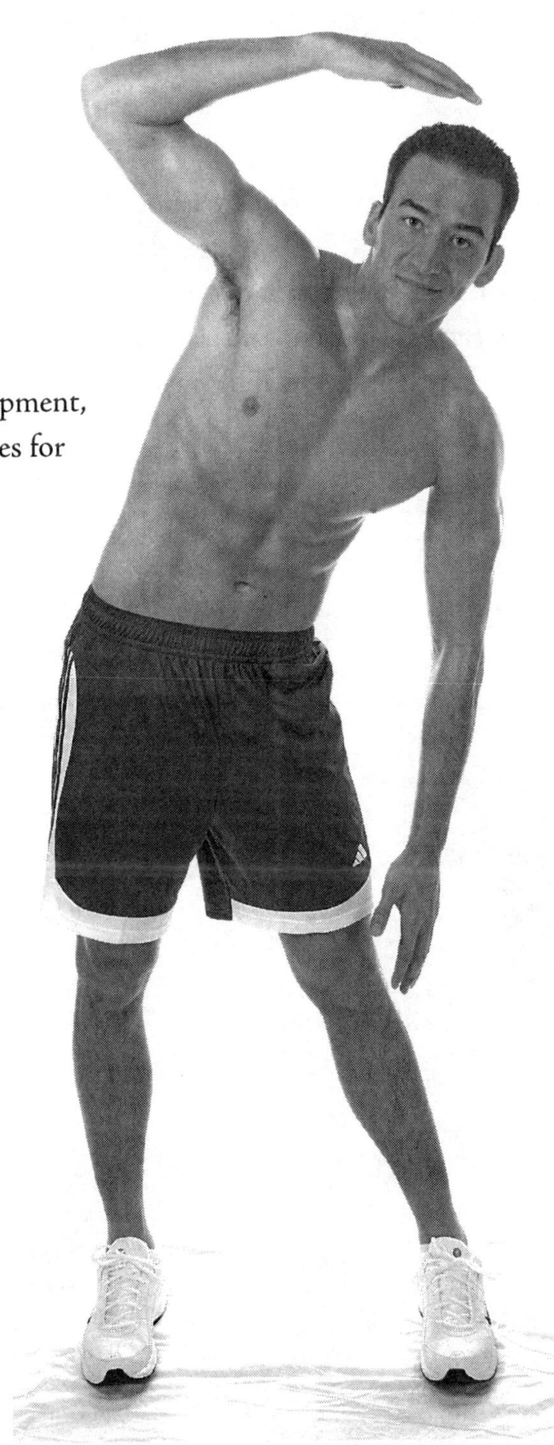

You can have strong, rippling washboard abs! No equipment, weights, pulleys, or machines! Just five simple PowerFlexes for 20 minutes a day.

Wild Workout® for Strong, Rippling Washboard Abs

A massively muscular chest combined with deeply rippled abdominal muscles is an impressive sight. The person possessing both will always attract interest. And envy!

With consistency, determination, and patience, it's possible to build strong, well-defined abdominal muscles more quickly than you'd believe. Strengthening your abdominal muscles will help you breathe more deeply, too, which will improve your general health.

No earthly creatures that I know of have stronger, more impressive abdominal muscles than the dolphin and the shark. Imagine the incredible strength it takes for a dolphin to pull itself out of the water and "walk" across it by balancing on its tail and flexing its abdominal muscles! Talk about functional strength! Sharks, on the other hand, don't do cute tricks for tourists. Their power, speed, and ferocity have inspired respect and terror for thousands of years. Now let's PowerFlex®!

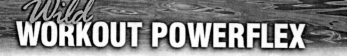

#1—DOLPHIN FLEX I

Dolphins swim by using their abdominal muscles to move their tail fins up and down. This PowerFlex® imitates that movement. Lie flat on the floor on your back (or on an exercise mat or carpet). Put your hands under your buttocks with your palms down. Your legs should be together and straight. Keeping your legs together and straight, lift them until they're pointing straight up. Then lower them to the floor again.

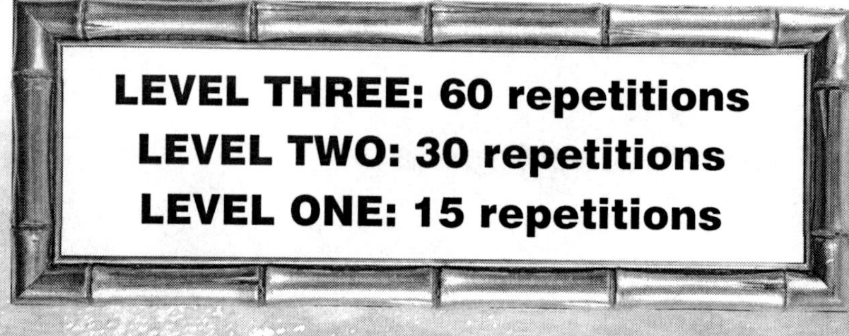

LEVEL THREE: 60 repetitions
LEVEL TWO: 30 repetitions
LEVEL ONE: 15 repetitions

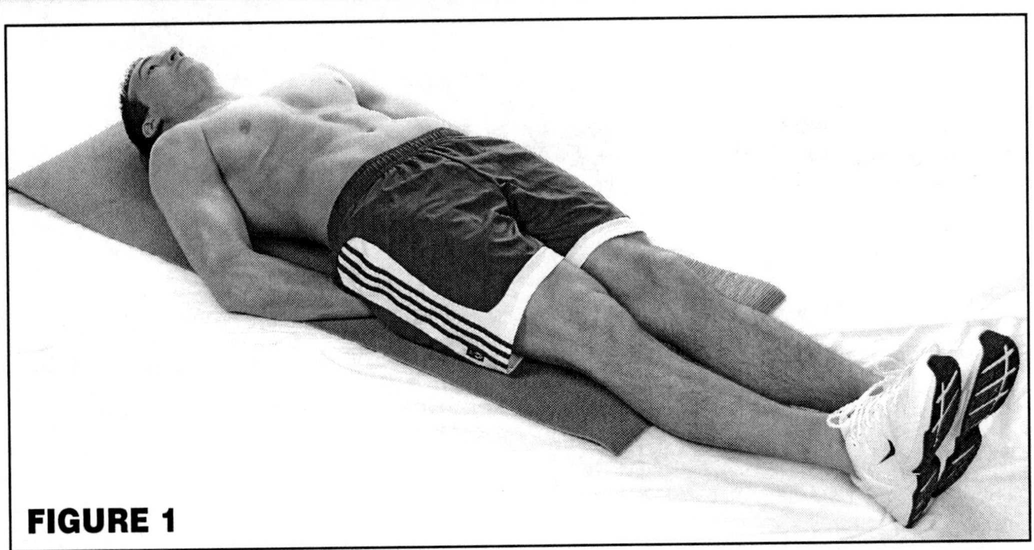

FIGURE 1

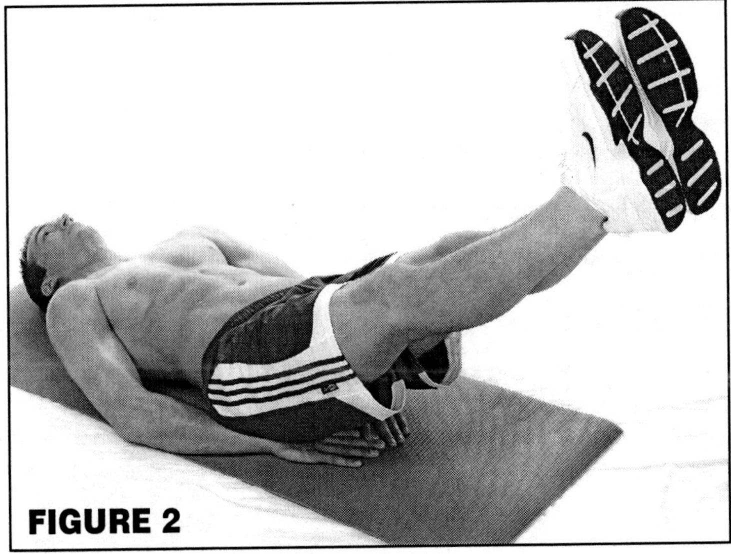

FIGURE 2

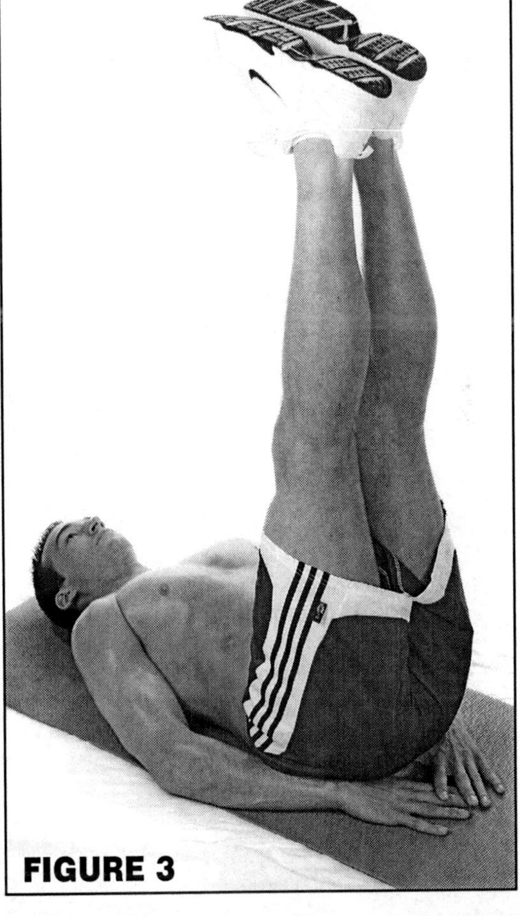

FIGURE 3

#2—DOLPHIN FLEX II

Lie flat on the floor on your back (or on an exercise mat or carpet). Keep your legs together and straight, resting the palms of your hands beside your ears. Tense your abdominal muscles and sit up as far as you can while keeping your legs on the floor. Try to touch your elbows to your knees. If you can, great. If you can't, that's okay—raise your body as far as you can without straining. This stimulates the stomach muscles, similar to the dolphin's movements.

This PowerFlex® is tough for most people—but then again, "most people" won't do the work necessary to build washboard abs. Patience and consistency are your keys. Exercise is like a bank account: you only get out of it what you put into it. And when you put a lot into it, expect to earn lots of interest!

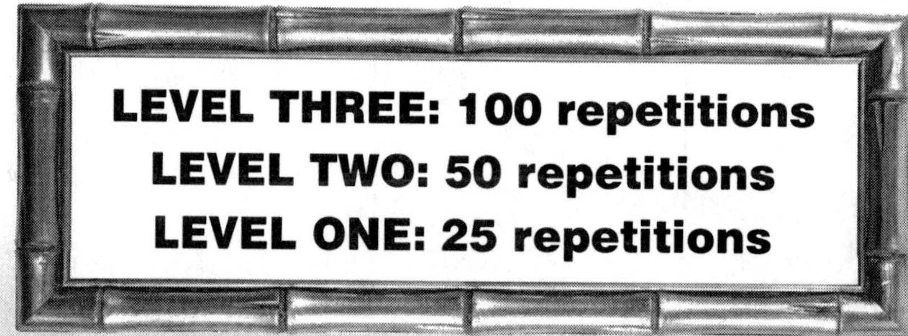

LEVEL THREE: 100 repetitions
LEVEL TWO: 50 repetitions
LEVEL ONE: 25 repetitions

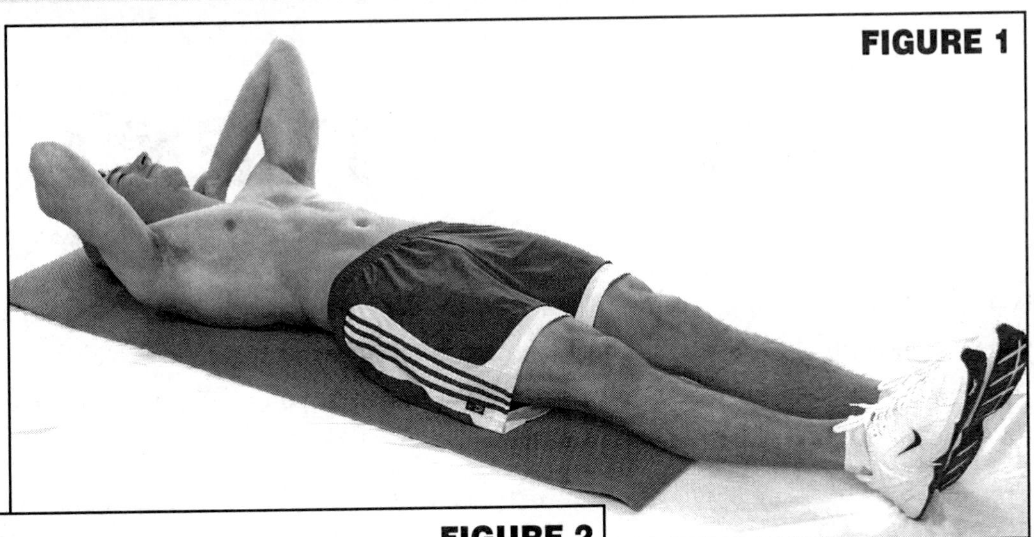
FIGURE 1

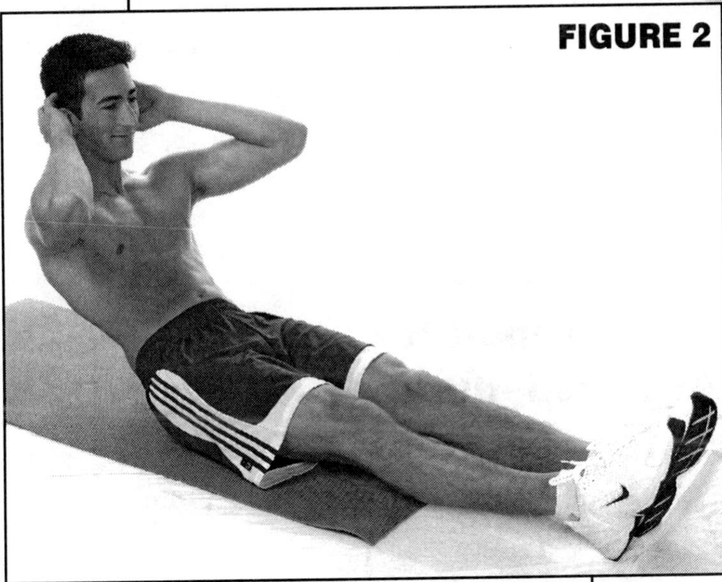
FIGURE 2

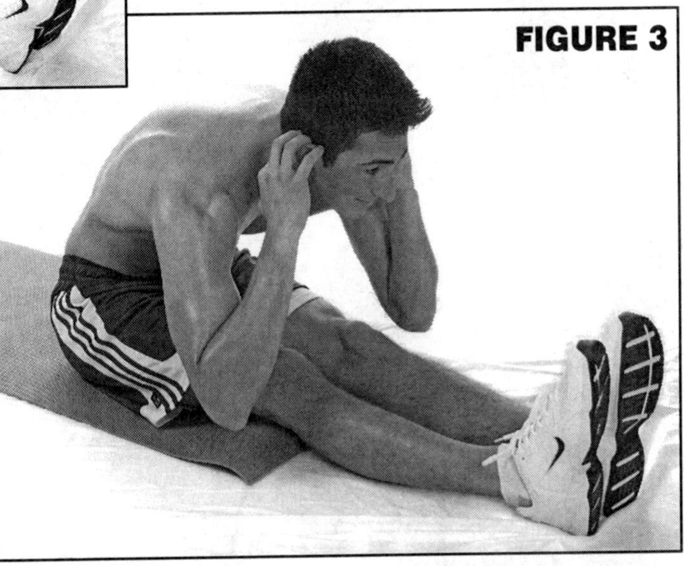
FIGURE 3

#3—SHARK FLEX I

Sharks don't act like dolphins, and they don't swim like them, either. While dolphins swim by moving their tails up and down, sharks swim by moving theirs from side to side. You need to do both up-and-down and side-to-side movements to strengthen your abdominal muscles from all angles—and to deepen all the ridges in your washboard!

Lie flat on the floor on your back (or on an exercise mat or carpet). Put your hands under your buttocks with your palms down. Lift your legs until they point straight up. Now, move your feet like the shark moves its fins. Open your legs until they form a wide V, then bring them back together and cross them. Your right foot will stretch toward the left and your left foot will stretch toward the right. It's a four-part movement: up, out, cross, and down. With each repetition, alternate which leg you cross in front.

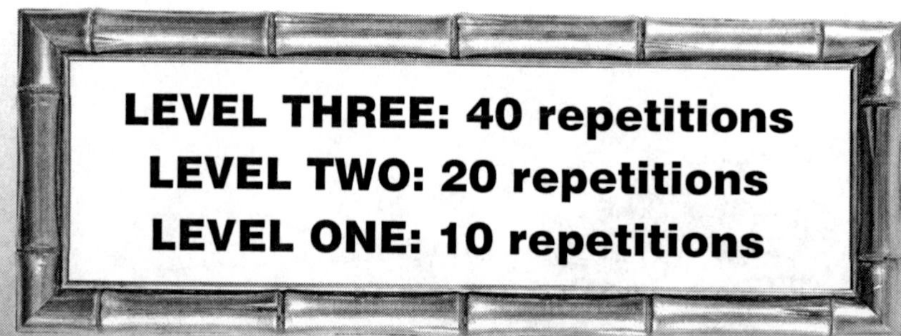
LEVEL THREE: 40 repetitions
LEVEL TWO: 20 repetitions
LEVEL ONE: 10 repetitions

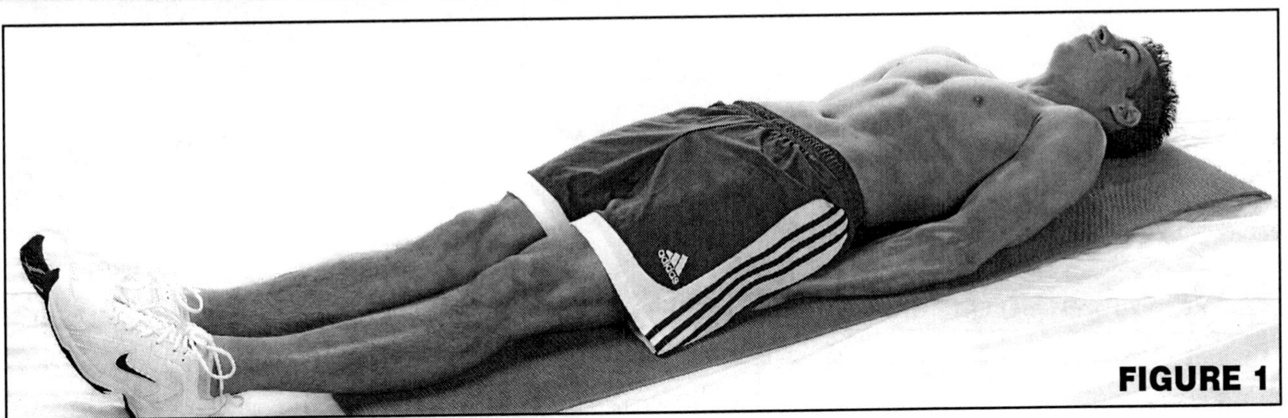

FIGURE 1

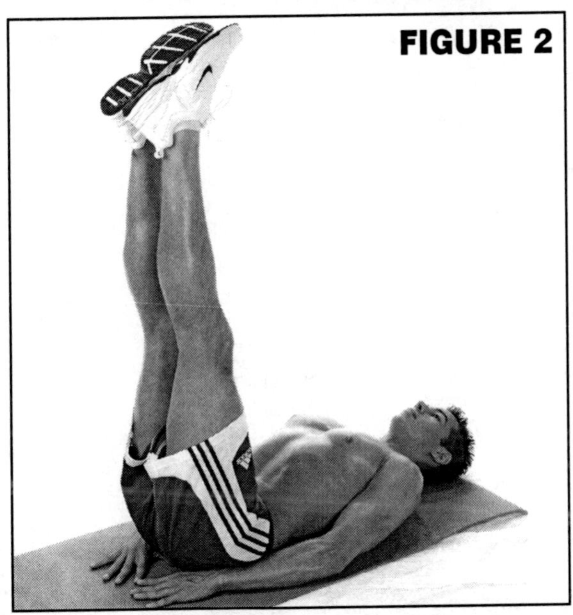

FIGURE 2

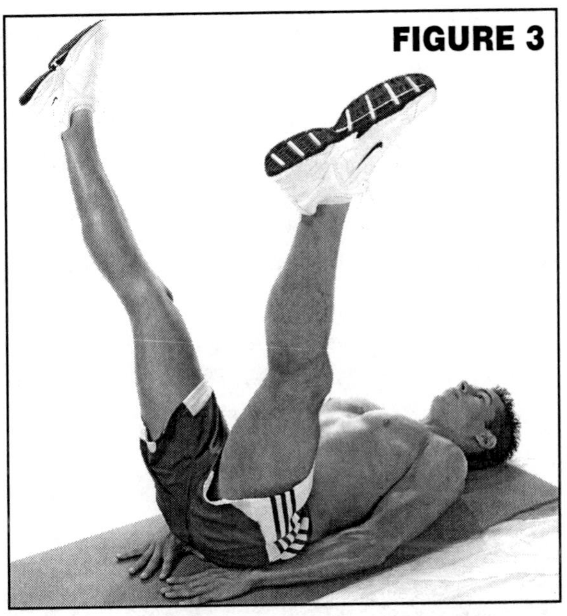

FIGURE 3

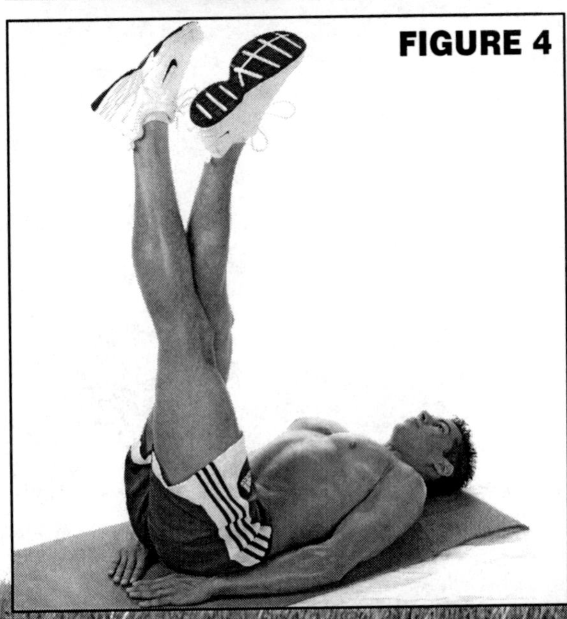

FIGURE 4

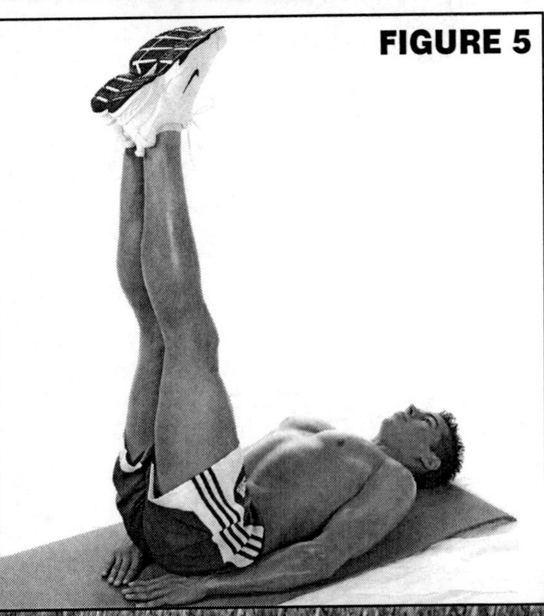

FIGURE 5

#4—SHARK FLEX II

We've all seen men and women walking around with "love handles"—bulges of unsightly fat hanging above their belts at their sides. This PowerFlex® targets the obliques, the muscles underneath those "love handles." You are going to simulate the shark's side-to-side movement with your upper body.

Stand with your hands on your hips, your feet shoulder-width apart, and your legs straight. Bend to your right as far as you can without straining. Let your right hand slide down your right leg as you bend. As your right hand slides down, curl your left arm upward until it's over your head and pointing to the right. Doing this will help you bend a little farther to the right. Return to the starting position and repeat, bending to your left this time. Again, don't stretch farther than is comfortable for you.

REMEMBER: Wild Workout® should feel good to do!

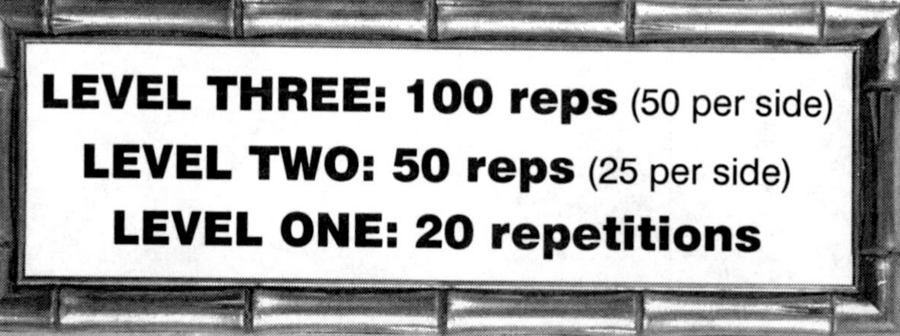

LEVEL THREE: 100 reps (50 per side)
LEVEL TWO: 50 reps (25 per side)
LEVEL ONE: 20 repetitions

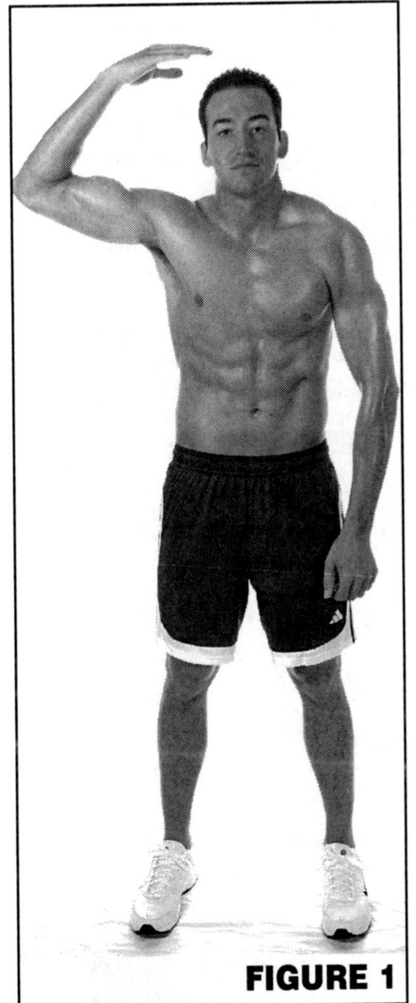

FIGURE 1

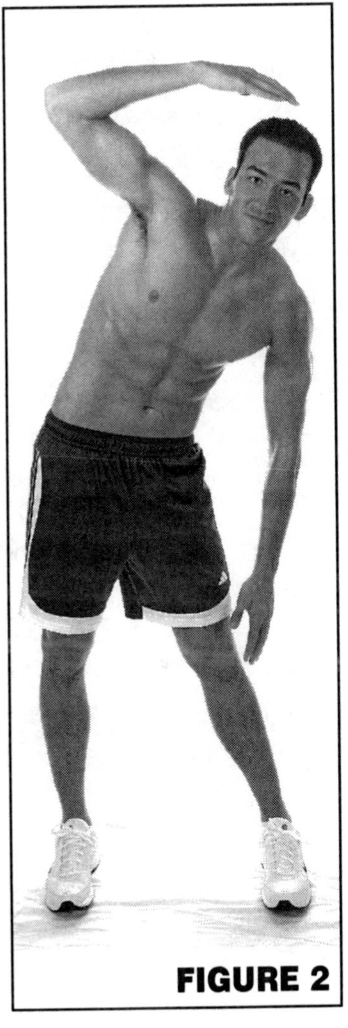

FIGURE 2

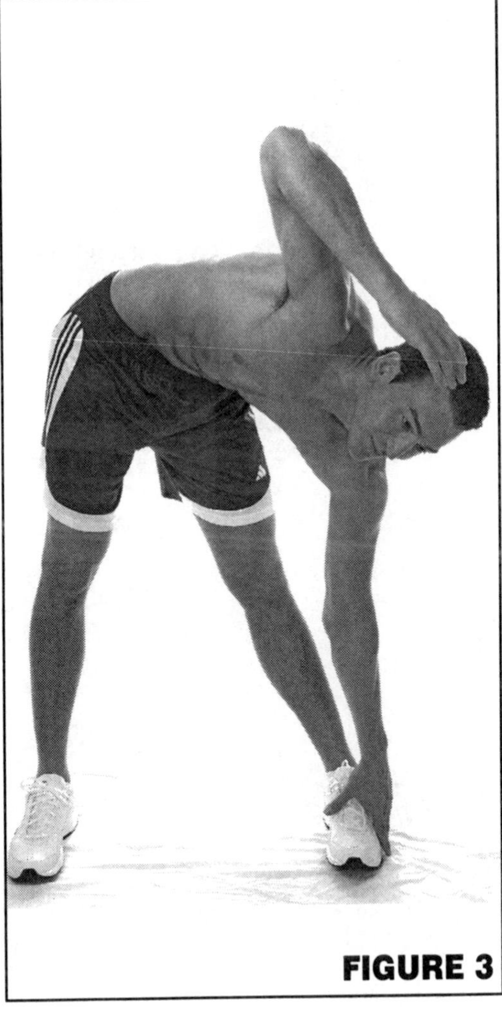

FIGURE 3

#5—DOLPHIN FLEX III

Here's one last up-and-down movement to finish your workout. First, set a sturdy chair or stool a few feet away from a heavy piece of furniture (such as a bed, dresser, or couch). Sit sideways on the chair or stool and slide your feet under the bed, dresser, or couch. Now that you're in position, rest the palms of your hands beside your ears and lean back slowly. If you can, lean back until your body's parallel to the floor. Then tense your abdominal muscles as you sit back up. Don't lean back farther than is comfortable for you and never bend past a 90° angle—to do so could hurt your lower back.

That's it, my friend. By practicing these five PowerFlexes regularly and eating sensibly, you'll build lean washboard abs where your belly used to be! Just to be clear, "eating sensibly" means eating lots of fresh vegetables and fruits, along with whole grains and lean meat. Be sure to drink plenty of water, too.

LEVEL THREE: 100 repetitions
LEVEL TWO: 50 repetitions
LEVEL ONE: 25 repetitions

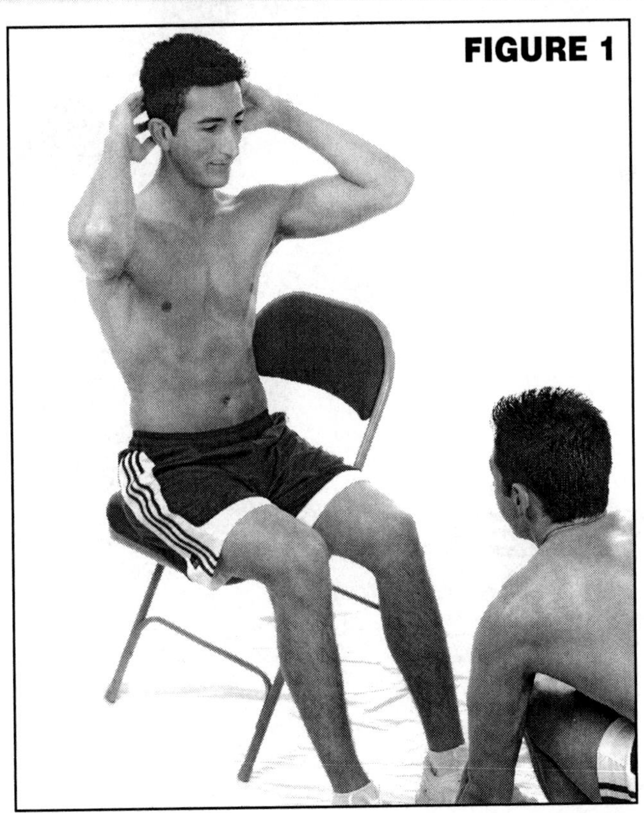
FIGURE 1

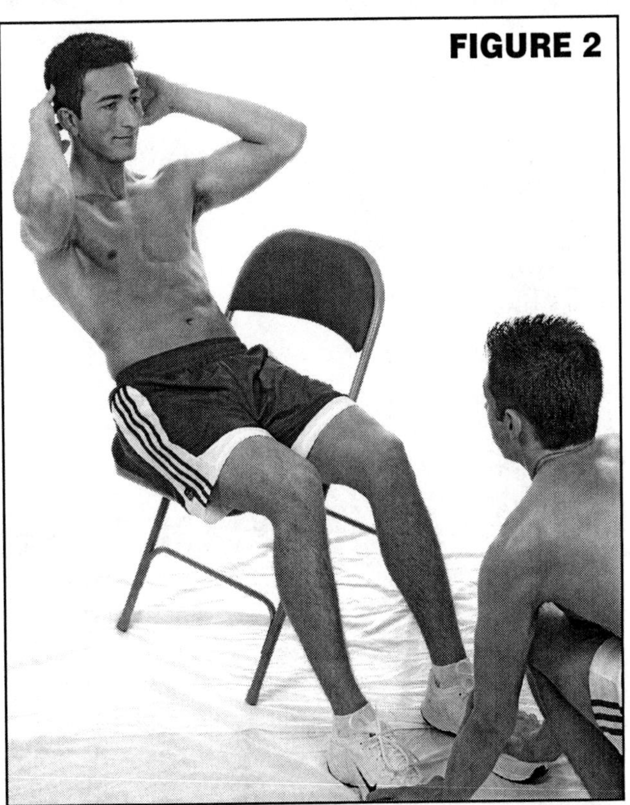
FIGURE 2

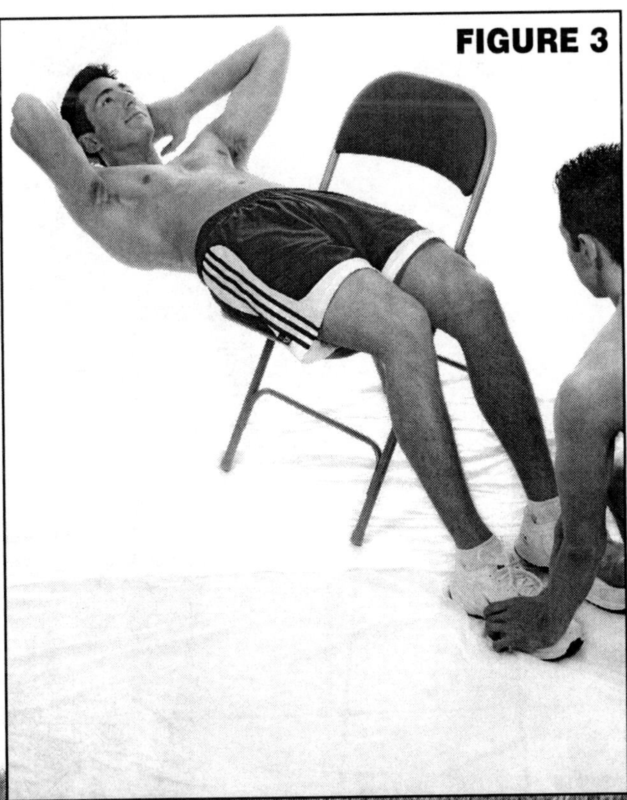
FIGURE 3

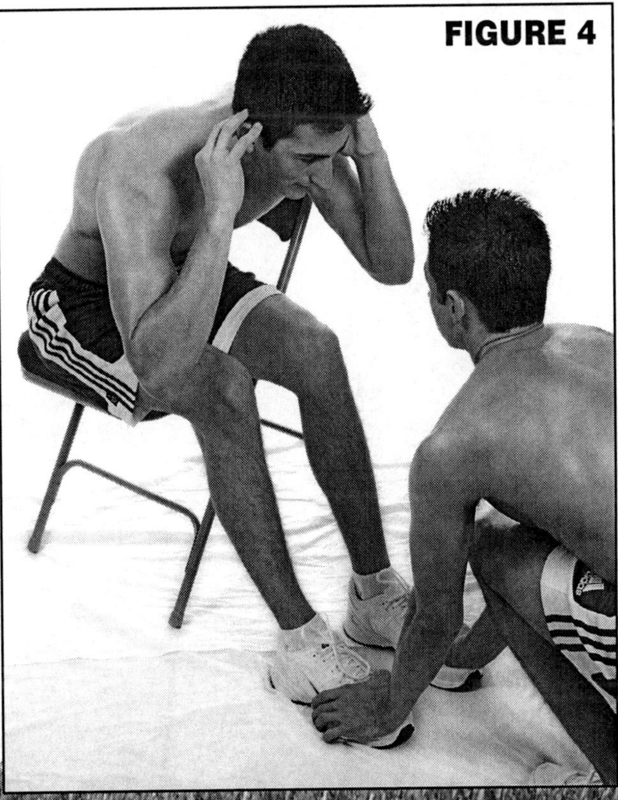
FIGURE 4

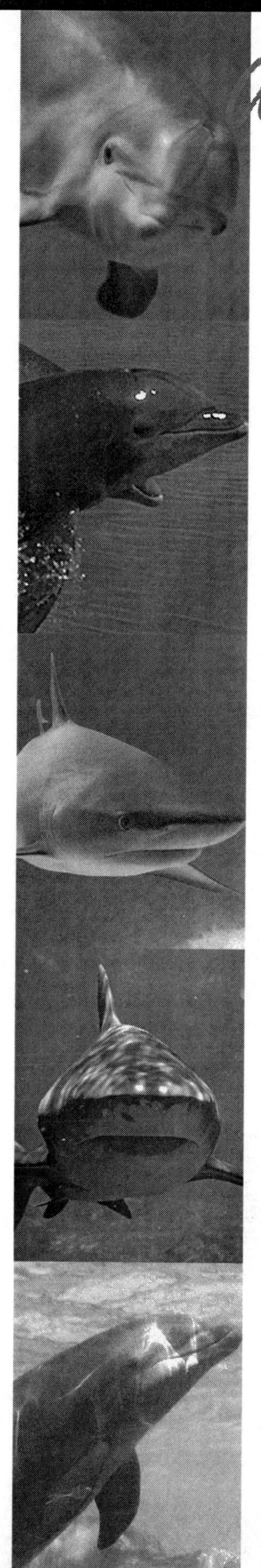

Abdominal Exercises

DOLPHIN FLEX I

DOLPHIN FLEX II

SHARK FLEX I

SHARK FLEX II

DOLPHIN FLEX III

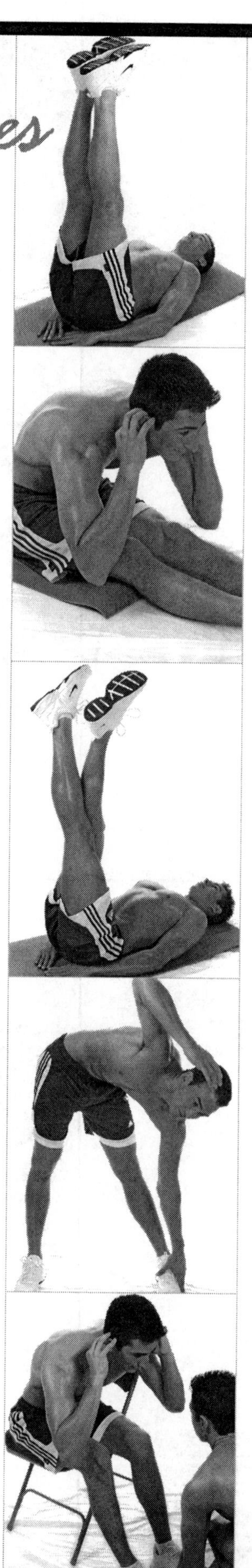

POWERFLEX *Spine*

SPINE WORKOUT

You can have a healthy, flexible, energetic spine without the use of special equipment, pulleys, or machines. Just do these five PowerFlexes for 20 minutes a day.

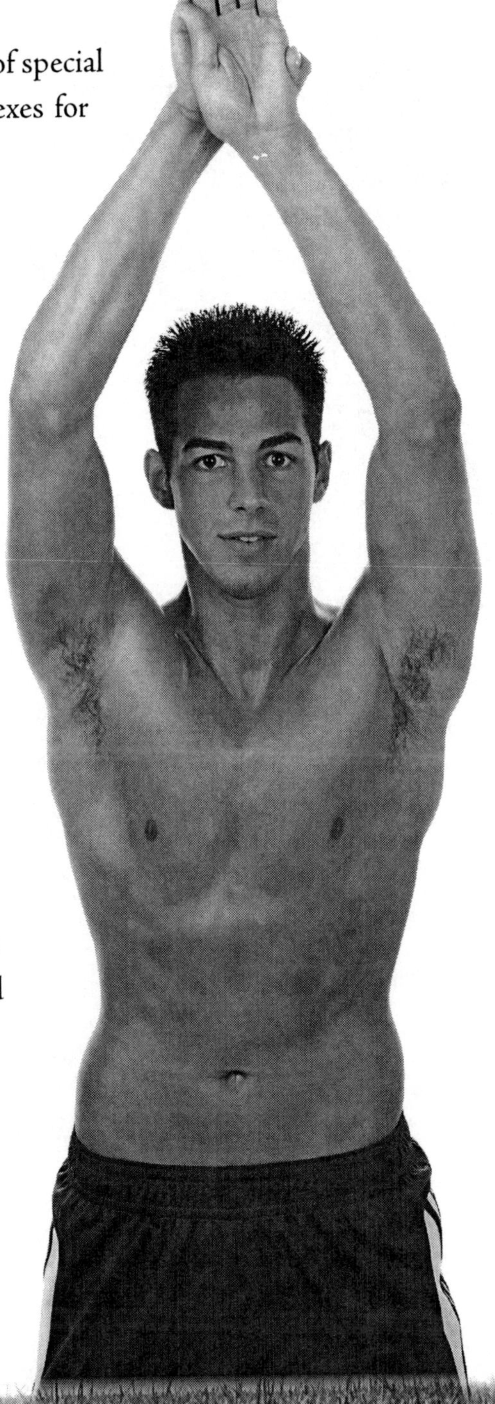

Wild Workout® for a Healthy, Flexible, Energetic Spine

Like a transformer tower that holds up ultra-high power electrical lines, the human spine holds up the spinal cord, which moves electrical energy—the vitality, radiance, and power of health—through the body. The spinal column is made up of 24 separate bones (or vertebrae) and two fused bones, the sacrum (with five bones) and the coccyx (with four bones). If any of these separate or fused bones is out of place, energy won't move through the body the way it's meant to. If energy becomes blocked, pain and illness often follow. Any chiropractor will tell you that your health—physical and mental—depends on the health and flexibility of your spine. Yet very few other exercise courses include movements designed to protect and improve the spine's health and flexibility. The five PowerFlexes in this Workout imitate the movements of the eel and the alligator, two creatures whose incredibly flexible spines allow them to twist, turn, swim, and strike with purpose and power.

IMPORTANT: Do the PowerFlexes in this workout slowly and smoothly. Don't bend or twist any farther than is comfortable for you and don't use high tension in your muscles when doing them. These PowerFlexes aren't as difficult as other ones you've done, but doing them will make all the other PowerFlexes more effective. Now, let's get WILD!

#1—EEL FLEX I

Sit on a chair or stool and fold your arms in front of you. Twist to the left from your waist as far as you can comfortably. Then return to your starting position and twist to your right. Move smoothly and take your time. Twisting to the left once and to the right once counts as one repetition.

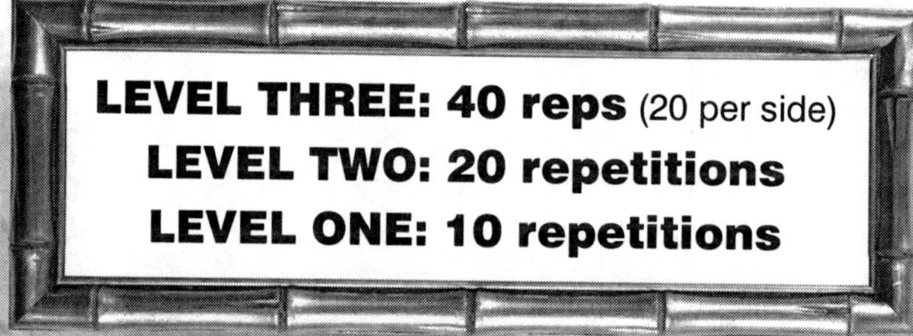

LEVEL THREE: 40 reps (20 per side)
LEVEL TWO: 20 repetitions
LEVEL ONE: 10 repetitions

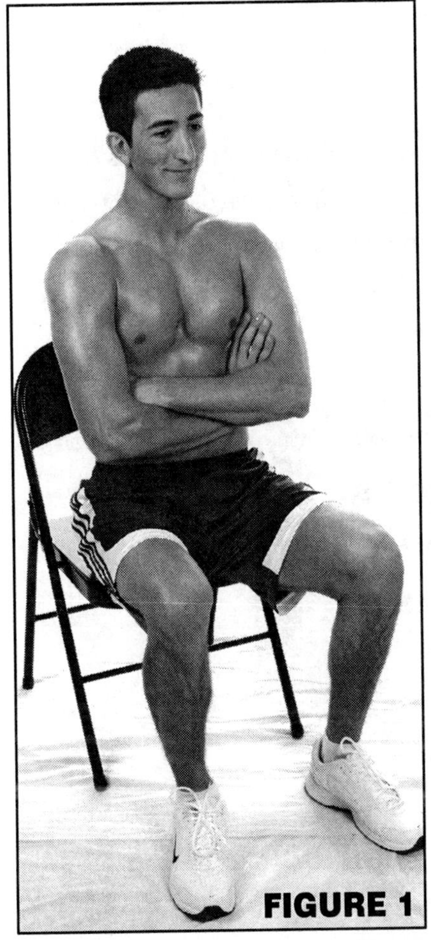
FIGURE 1

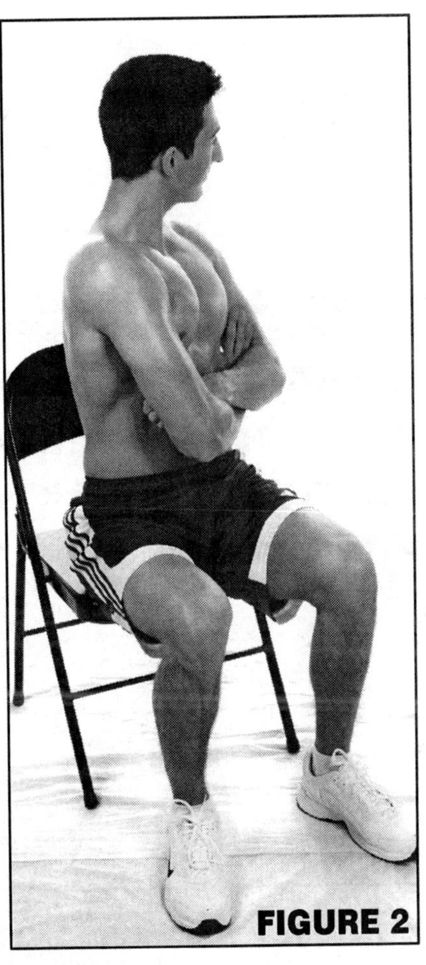
FIGURE 2

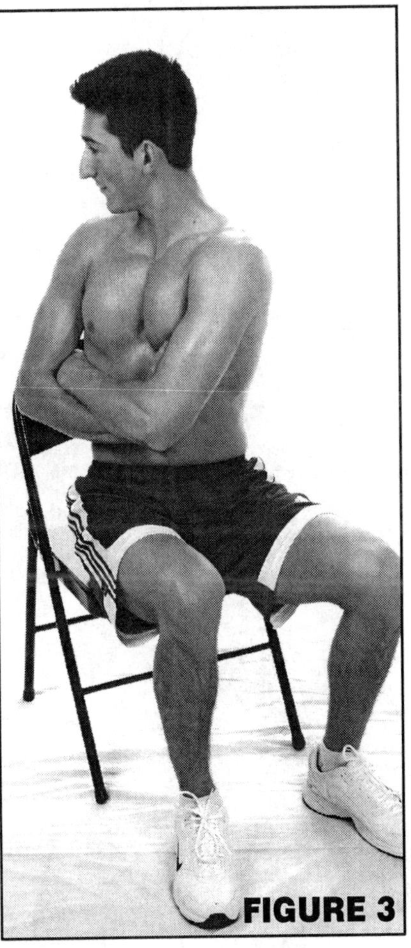
FIGURE 3

#2—EEL FLEX II

This Wild Workout® is for the upper part of the spine. While these exercises may not seem as strenuous as others, they are critical in keeping a flexible spine. Sit or stand facing forward and bend your head down as far as you can comfortably. Try to touch your chin to the bottom of your neck. Now, move your head back as far as you can comfortably. Try to touch the back of your head to the back of your neck. Again, move smoothly. Bending forward once and back once counts as one repetition.

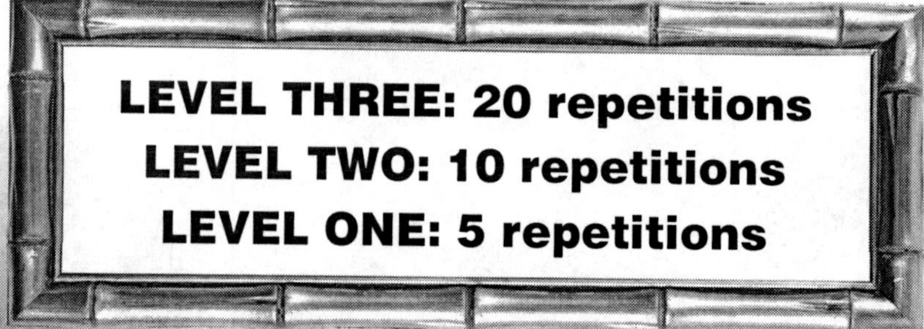

LEVEL THREE: 20 repetitions
LEVEL TWO: 10 repetitions
LEVEL ONE: 5 repetitions

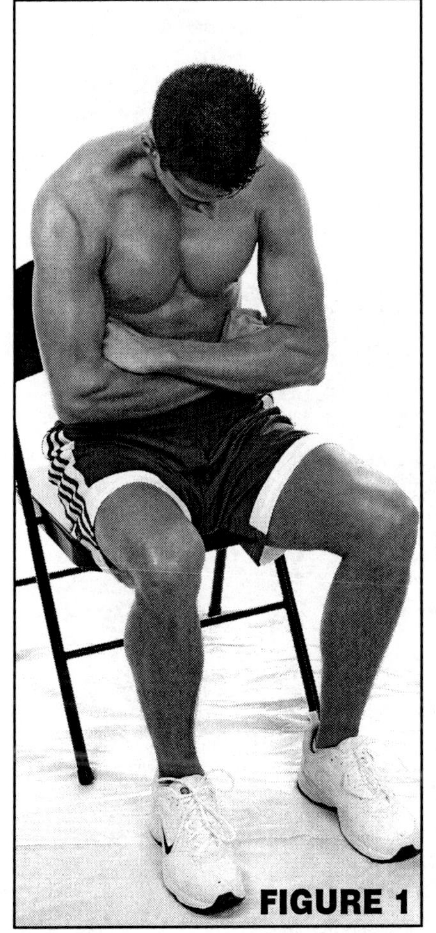
FIGURE 1

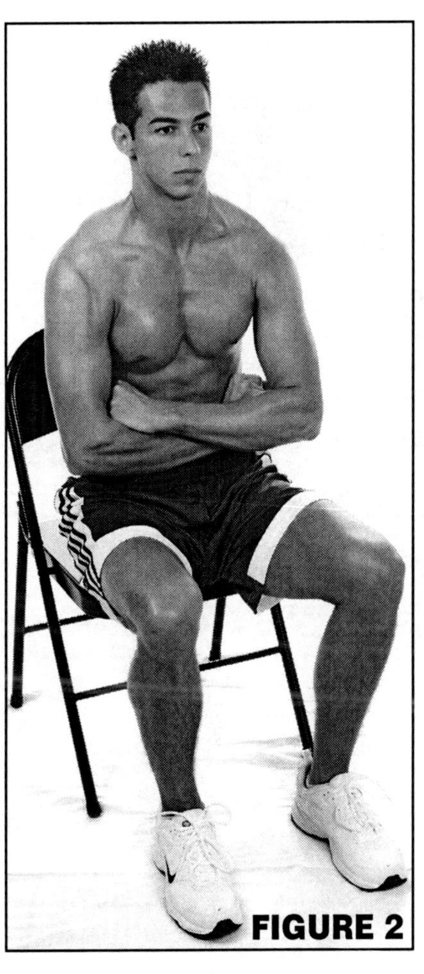
FIGURE 2

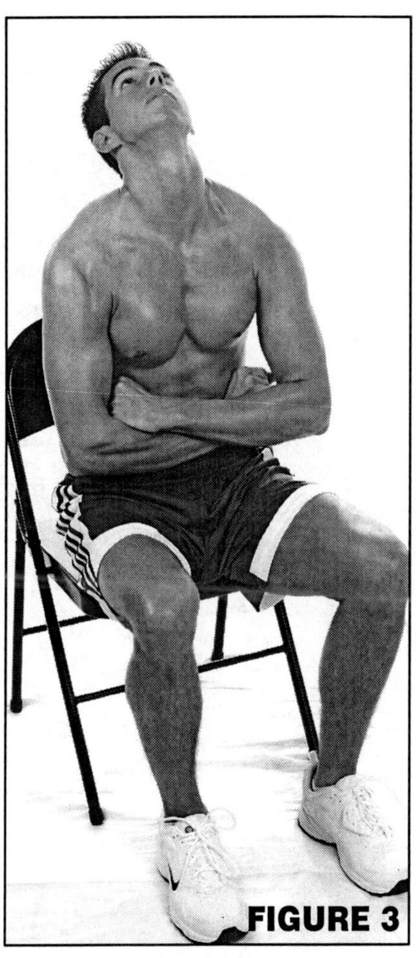
FIGURE 3

#3—ALLIGATOR FLEX I

The alligator is one of nature's greatest wrestlers, and its best move is the Alligator Roll. Thanks to its flexible spine, it can pull victims toward it by rolling its body. If you don't want to become a victim of back pain, be sure to do this PowerFlex®!

Stand with your feet shoulder-width apart. Clasp your hands behind your back and twist to your right as far as you can comfortably. Then repeat the movement while twisting to your left. Twisting to your right once and to your left once counts as one repetition.

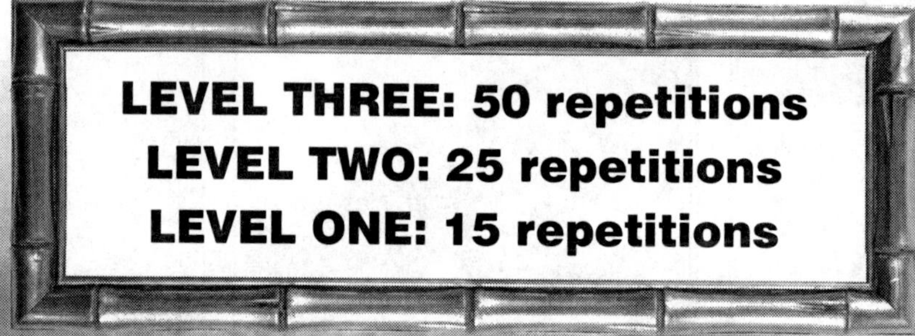

LEVEL THREE: 50 repetitions
LEVEL TWO: 25 repetitions
LEVEL ONE: 15 repetitions

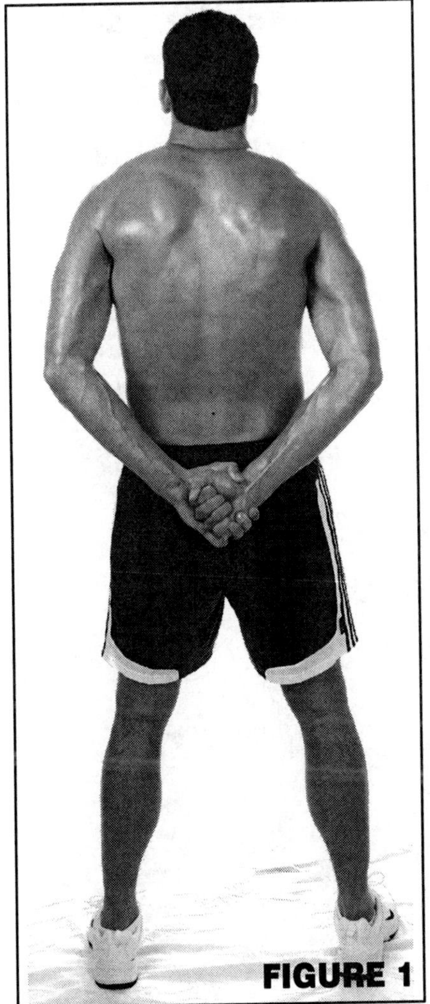

FIGURE 1

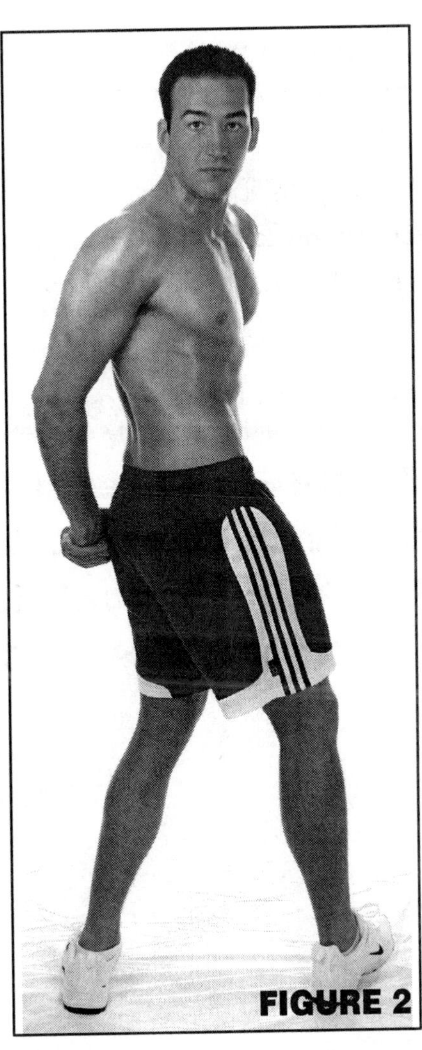

FIGURE 2

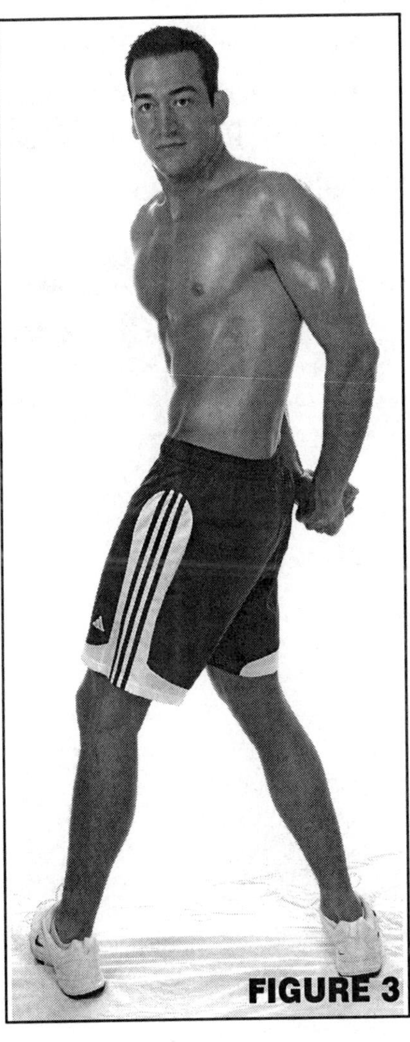

FIGURE 3

#4—ALLIGATOR FLEX II

This PowerFlex® stretches your spine in two ways, with a forward bend and a backward bend. This combination stimulates the movement of energy—and health— through the spine and throughout the body.

Stand with your feet together and your knees straight. Lift your arms overhead, then bend forward as far as you can comfortably while keeping your knees straight. Stand up again smoothly, raising your hands overhead again and bending backward. Don't try to bend backward farther than is comfortable for you.

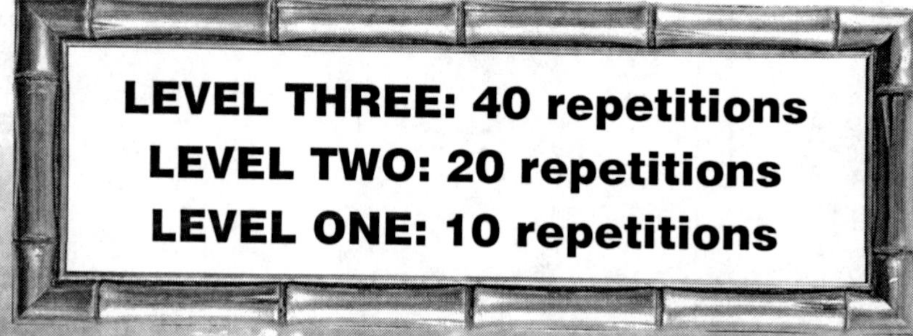

LEVEL THREE: 40 repetitions
LEVEL TWO: 20 repetitions
LEVEL ONE: 10 repetitions

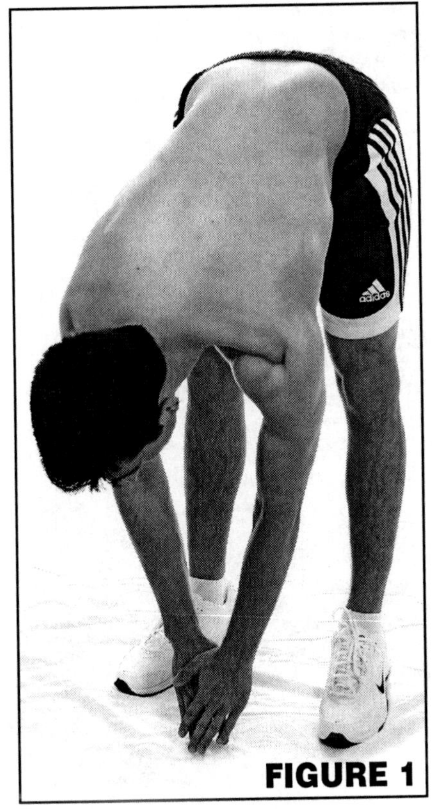
FIGURE 1

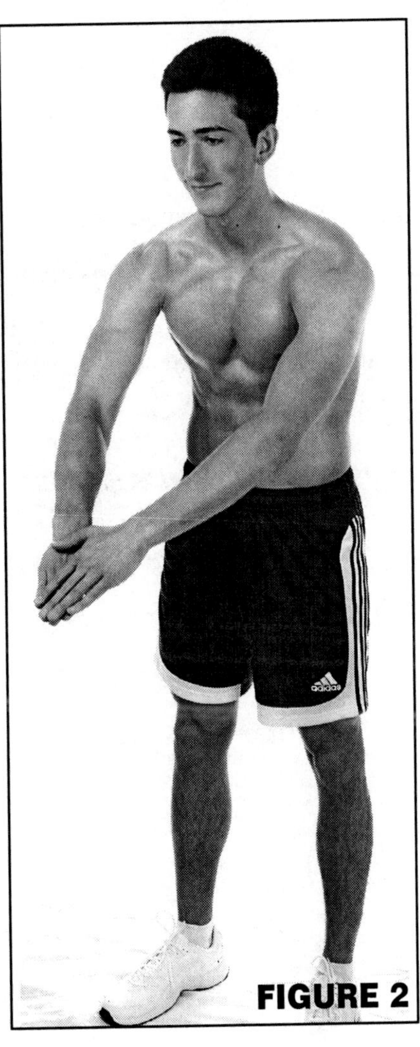
FIGURE 2

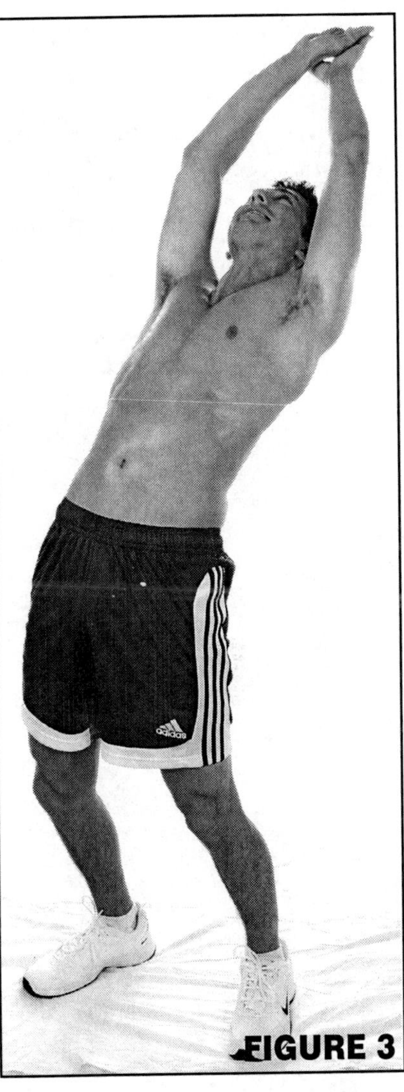
FIGURE 3

#5—EEL FLEX III

As you notice the eel has no hands, arms, feet or legs. It keeps fit and full of energy by twisting, turning, flexing, swimming, striking, all with its body's trunk. We are working out our spine the same way.

Stand with your feet together, your knees straight, and your arms straight overhead. Twist from the waist as far as you can to your left, then twist as far as you can to the right.

There you are, friend. Practicing these PowerFlexes consistently and patiently will go a long way toward protecting and improving your spine's health. Always remember that your mental and physical health depend on the health and flexibility of your spine. After all, if you want to show "backbone," you'd better have a healthy one! Now get busy!

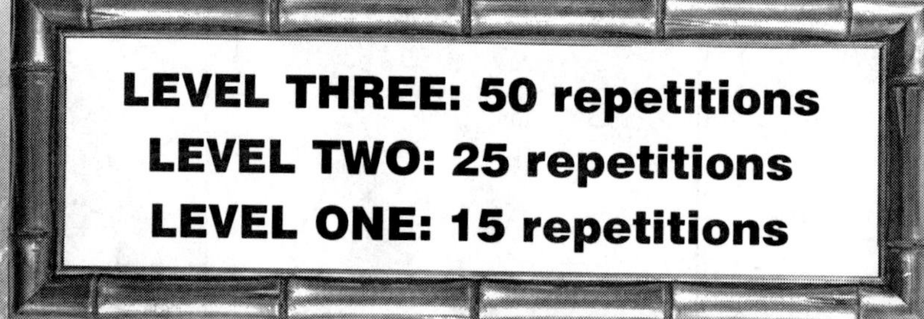

LEVEL THREE: 50 repetitions
LEVEL TWO: 25 repetitions
LEVEL ONE: 15 repetitions

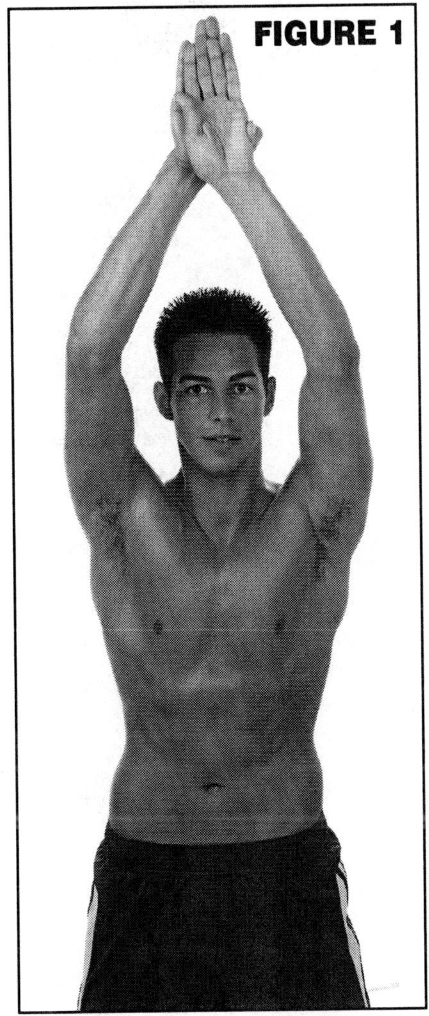
FIGURE 1

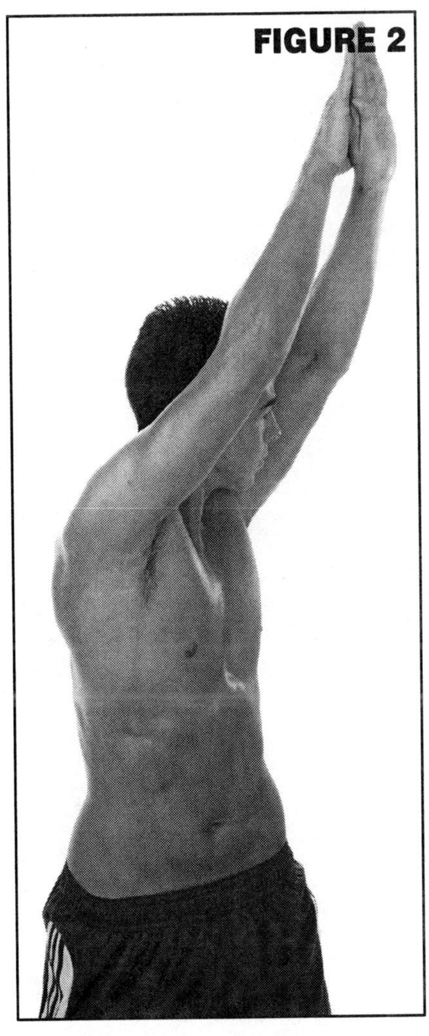
FIGURE 2

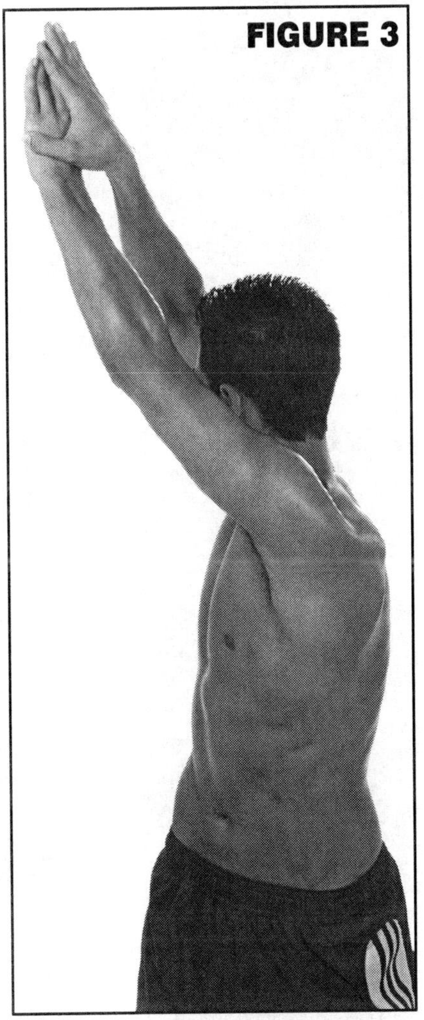
FIGURE 3

Spine Exercises

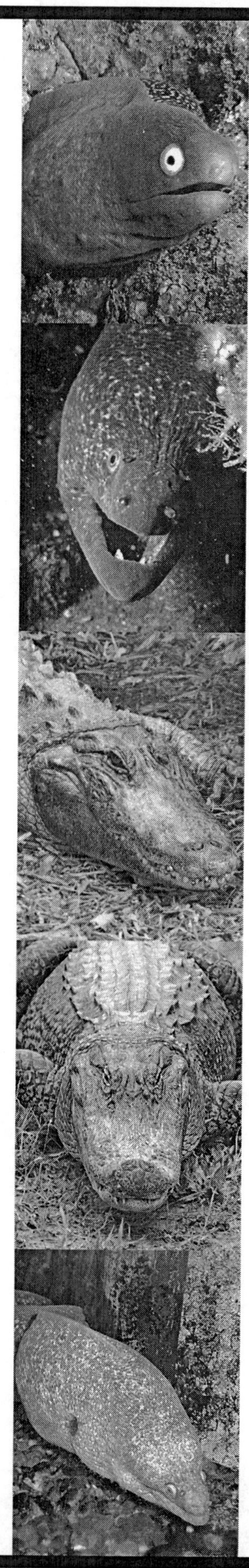

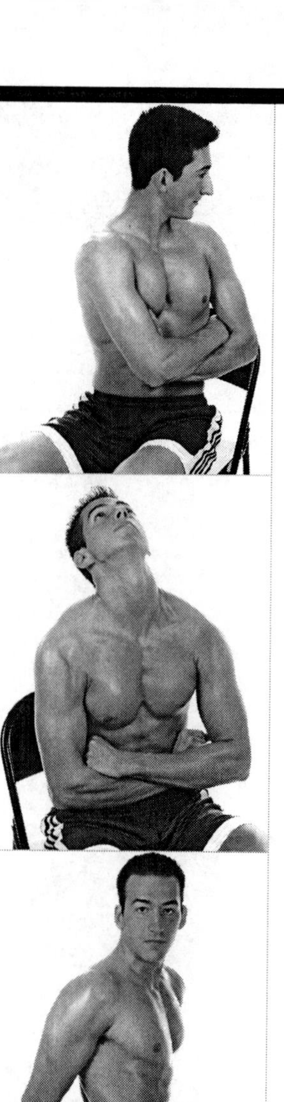

EEL FLEX I

EEL FLEX II

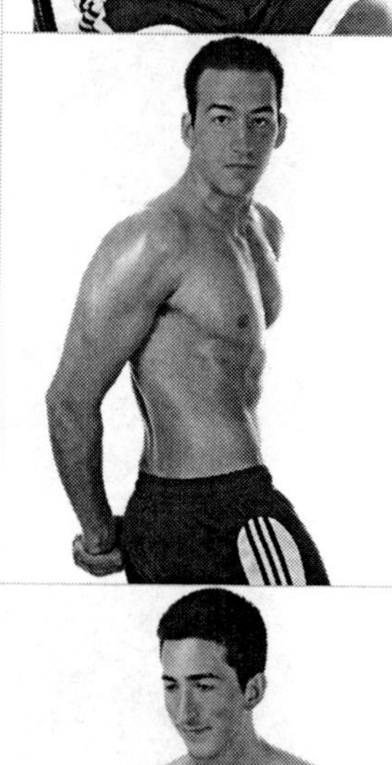

ALLIGATOR FLEX I

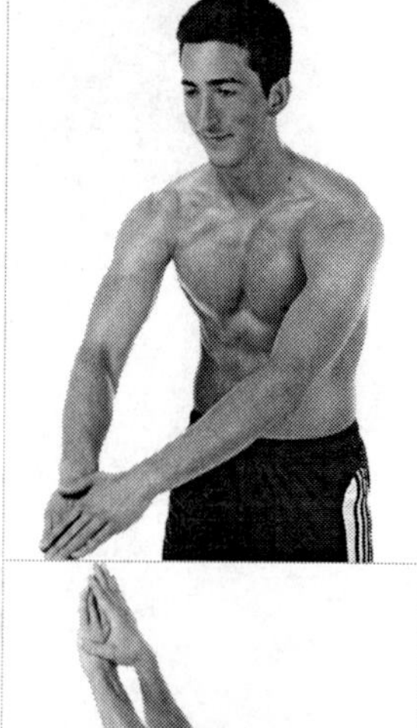

ALLIGATOR FLEX II

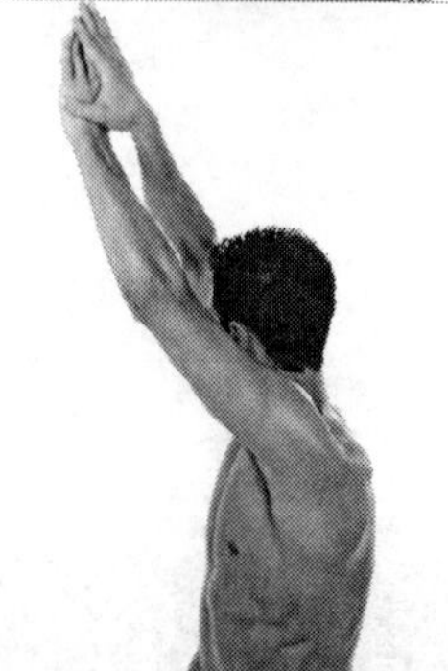

EEL FLEX III

POWERFLEX *Neck*

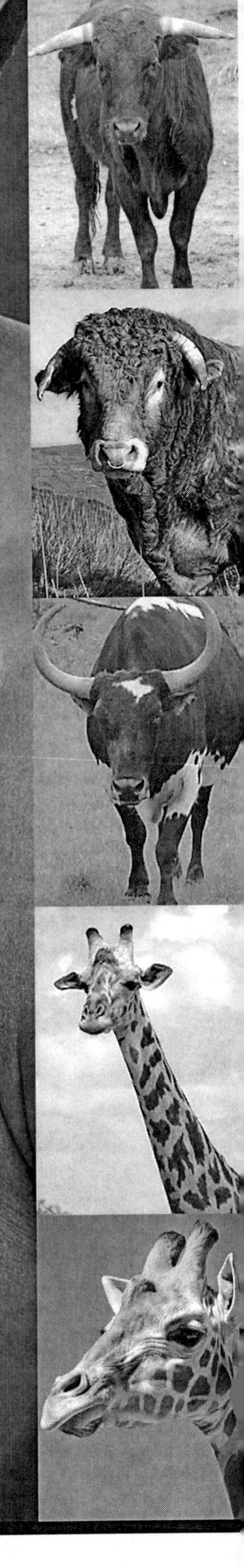

NECK WORKOUT

You can have a firm, strong, powerful neck without using equipment, weights, pulleys, or machines. Just do five PowerFlexes for 20 minutes a day.

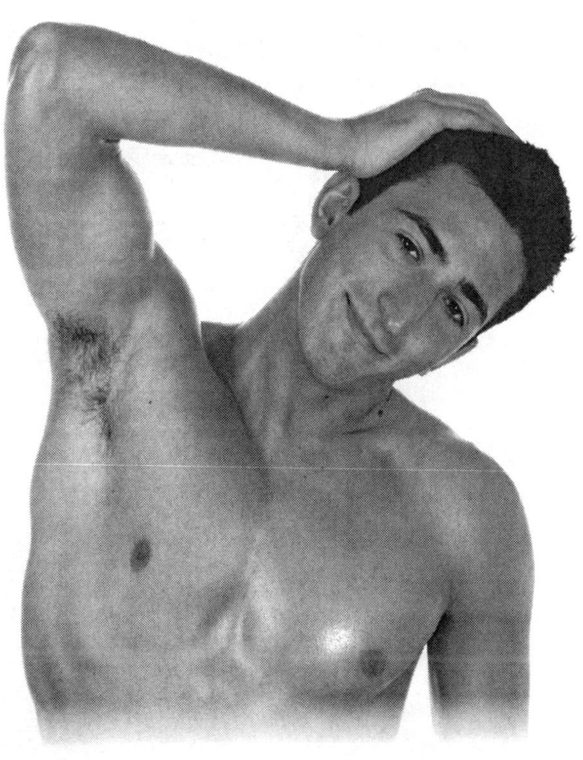

Wild Workout® for a Firm, Strong, Powerful Neck

You've probably heard tragic stories about athletes whose careers—or even lives—were ended by catastrophic neck injuries. Still, you don't have to be an athlete to suffer a neck injury. Just ask a car accident victim with whiplash. But whether you're a football player or martial artist, or whether you just share the road with tailgating drivers, the PowerFlexes in this workout can help you build a strong, muscular neck that's both injury-resistant and attractive.

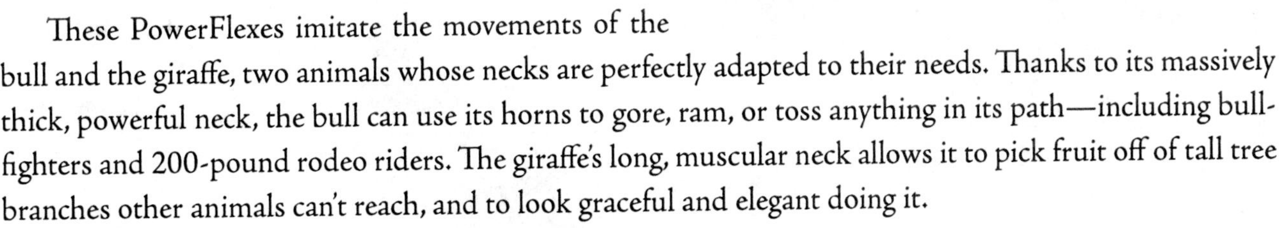

These PowerFlexes imitate the movements of the bull and the giraffe, two animals whose necks are perfectly adapted to their needs. Thanks to its massively thick, powerful neck, the bull can use its horns to gore, ram, or toss anything in its path—including bullfighters and 200-pound rodeo riders. The giraffe's long, muscular neck allows it to pick fruit off of tall tree branches other animals can't reach, and to look graceful and elegant doing it.

IMPORTANT: For four of the five PowerFlexes here, you'll use one of your hands to provide resistance. To avoid injury and sore muscles as you get started, keep the resistance light. Never force your neck, and remember to breathe as you do the movements. Now, let's get WILD!

#1—BULL FLEX I

This PowerFlex® works the muscles toward the front of the neck. Sit or stand, facing forward. Bend your head back as far as you can without straining. Place the palm of either hand on your forehead. Slowly and smoothly straighten your neck as you resist with your hand.

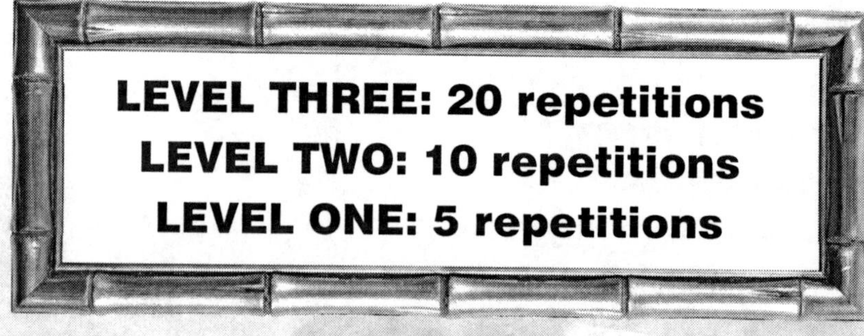

LEVEL THREE: 20 repetitions
LEVEL TWO: 10 repetitions
LEVEL ONE: 5 repetitions

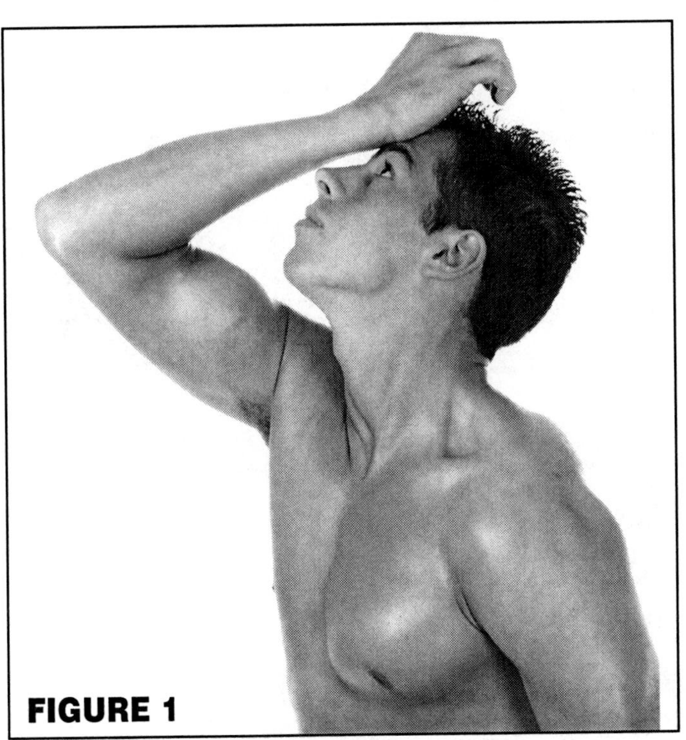

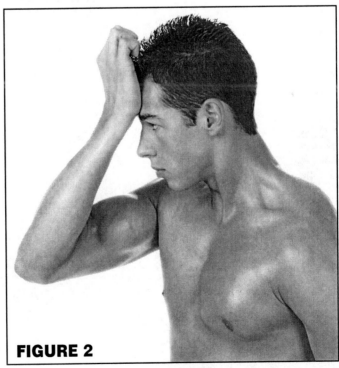

FIGURE 1

FIGURE 2

#2—BULL FLEX II

This PowerFlex® works the muscles toward the back of the neck. Sit or stand, facing forward. Bow your head forward as far as you can without straining. Place the palm of either hand against the back of your head. Slowly and smoothly straighten your neck as you resist with your hand.

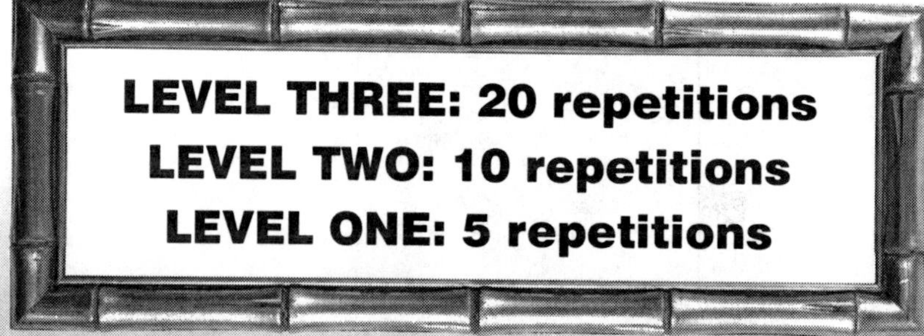

LEVEL THREE: 20 repetitions
LEVEL TWO: 10 repetitions
LEVEL ONE: 5 repetitions

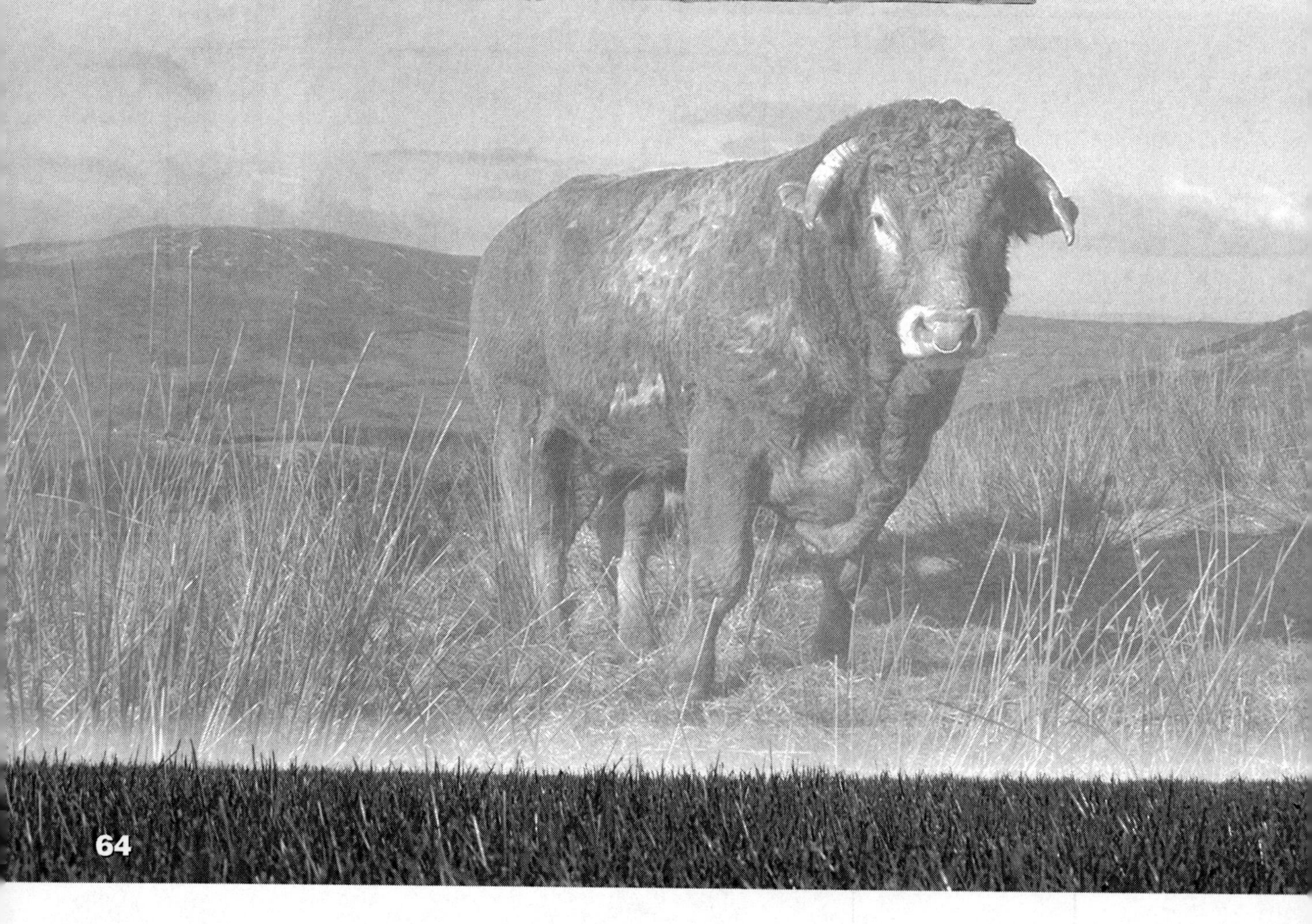

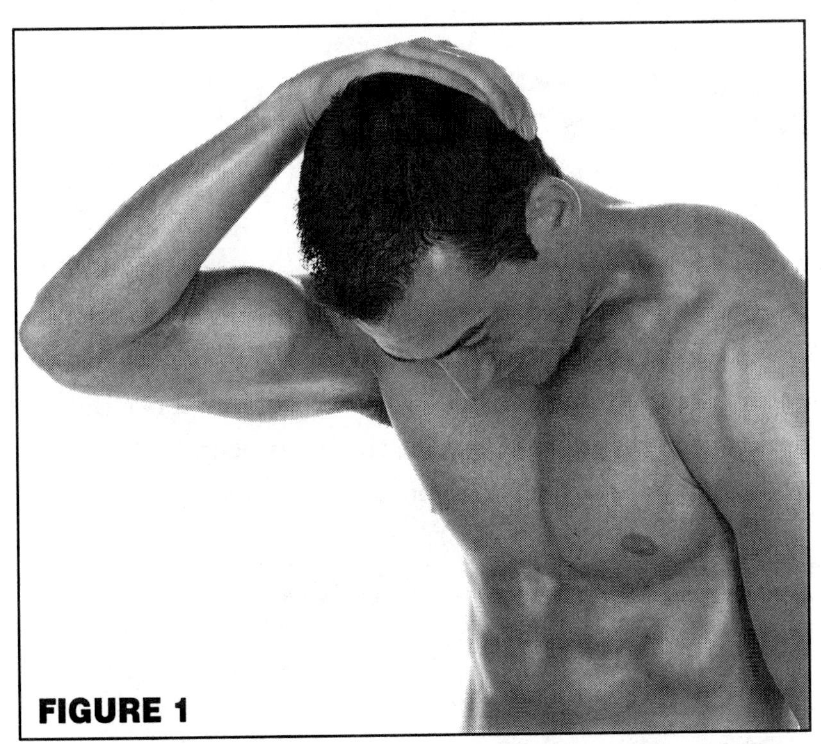

FIGURE 1

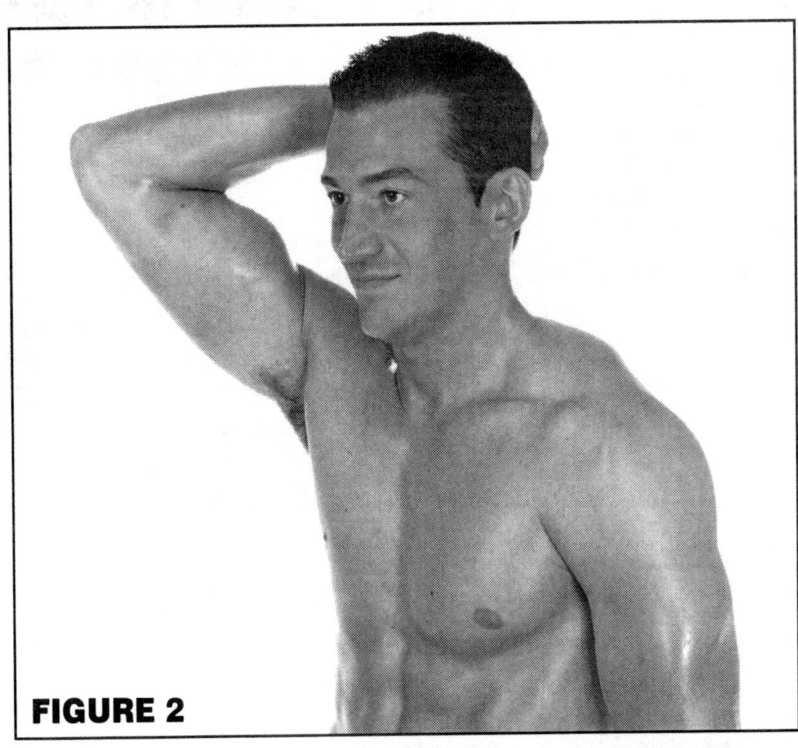

FIGURE 2

#3—BULL FLEX III

The next two PowerFlexes work the muscles along the sides of the neck. If you want to build a neck that's strong and attractive, it's very important to work your neck through its complete range of motion. Sit or stand, facing forward. Bow your head down and to the right as far as you can without straining. Place the palm of your left hand on the left side of your head, just above the ear. Slowly and smoothly straighten your neck as you resist. Then reverse the movement, bowing your head down and left and resisting with your right hand as you straighten your neck again.

LEVEL THREE: 40 reps (20 per side)
LEVEL TWO: 20 repetitions
LEVEL ONE: 10 repetitions

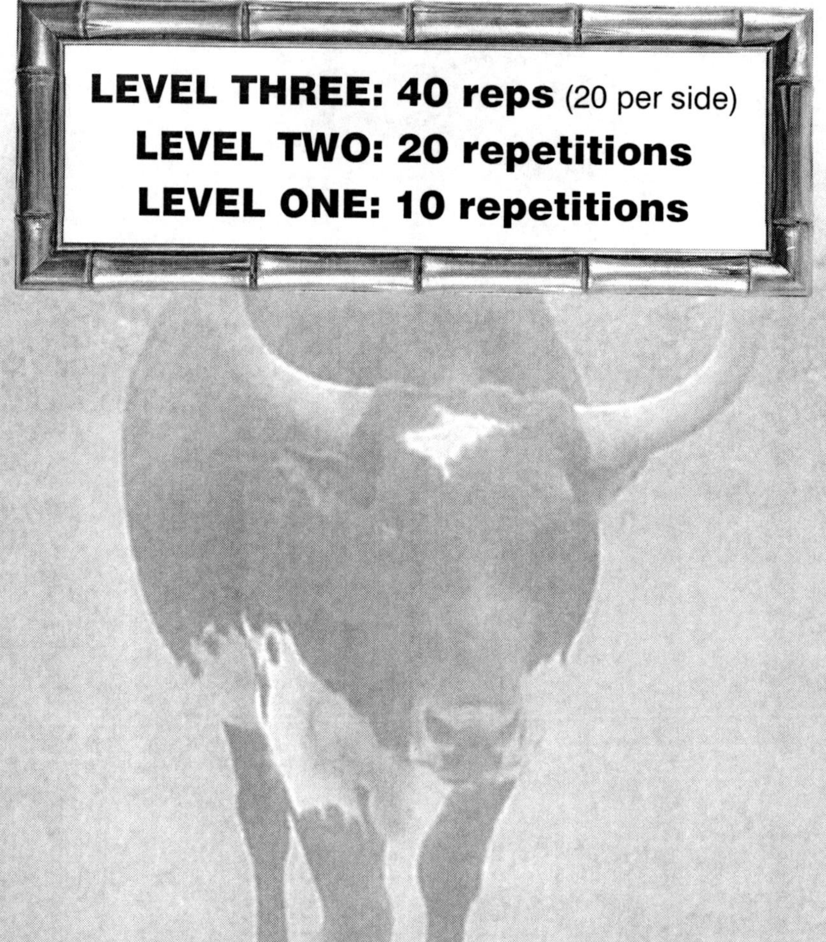

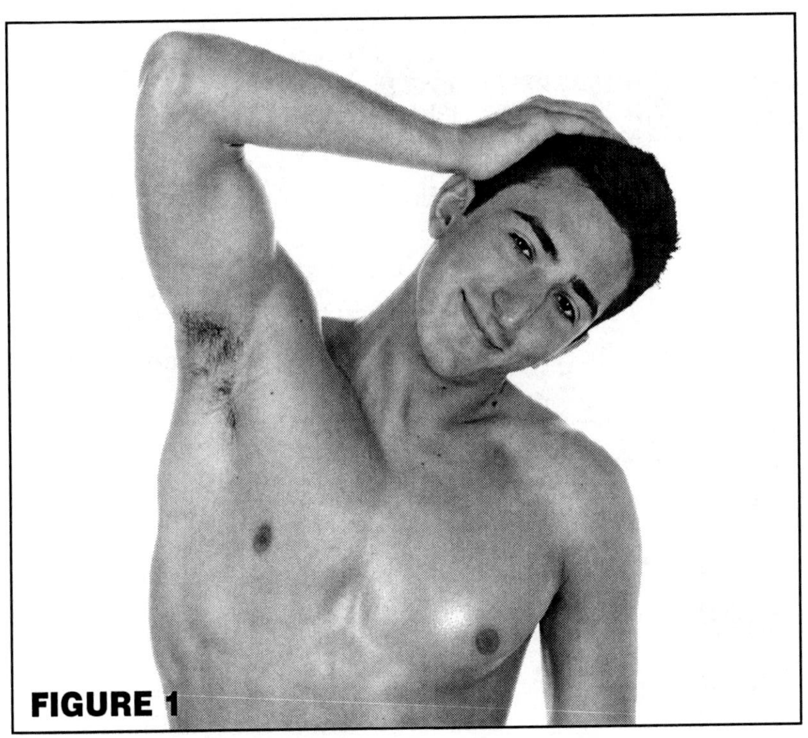
FIGURE 1

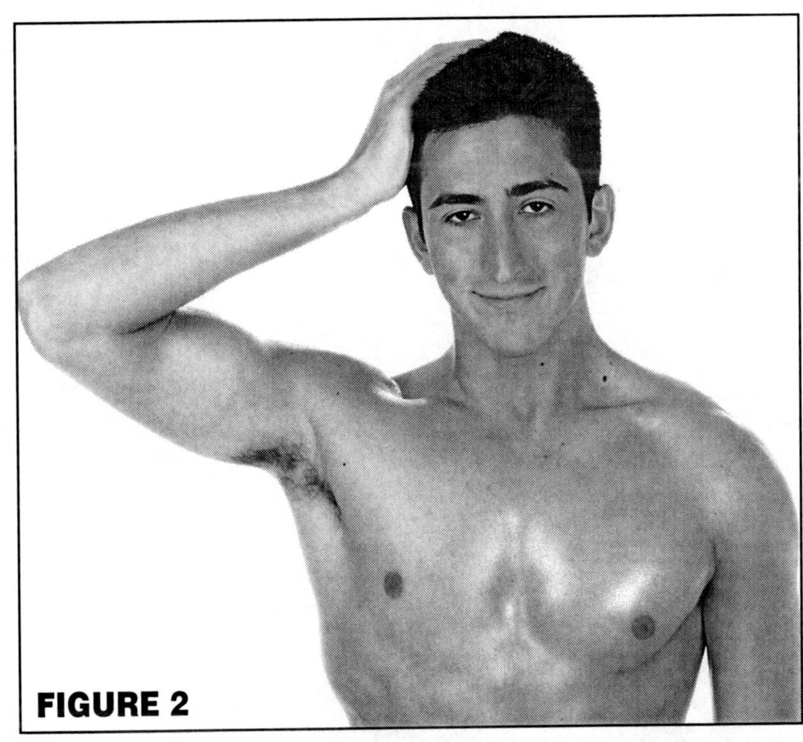
FIGURE 2

#4—GIRAFFE FLEX I

Sit or stand, facing forward. Keeping your neck straight, turn your head to the left. Place your right palm on the right side of your forehead. Slowly and smoothly turn your head, resisting with your right hand, until you're facing forward again. Switch hands and reverse the movement.

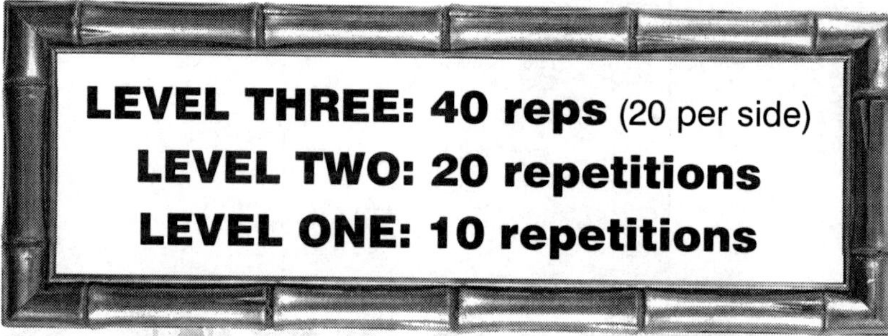

LEVEL THREE: 40 reps (20 per side)
LEVEL TWO: 20 repetitions
LEVEL ONE: 10 repetitions

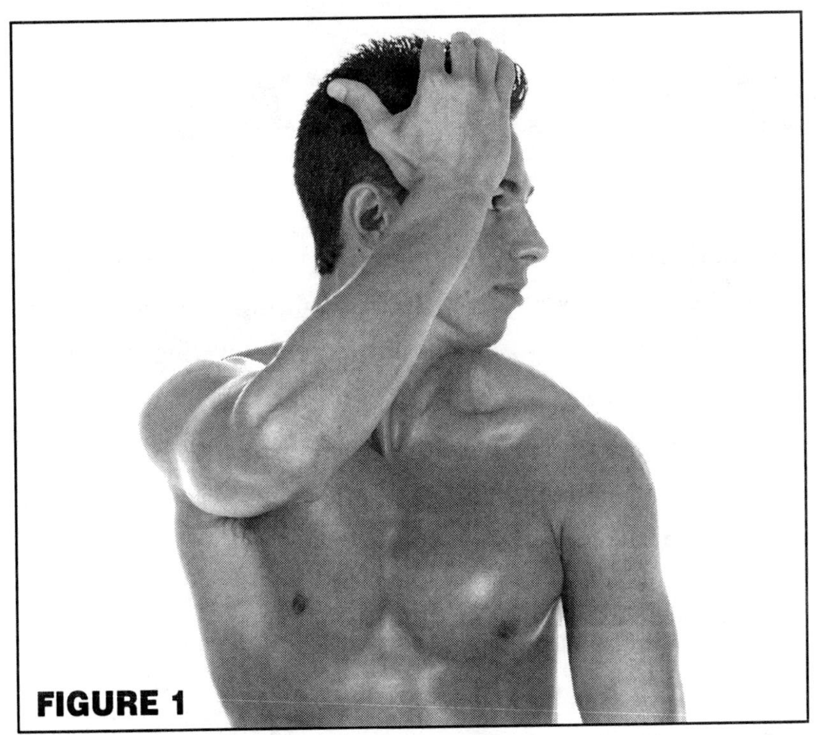
FIGURE 1

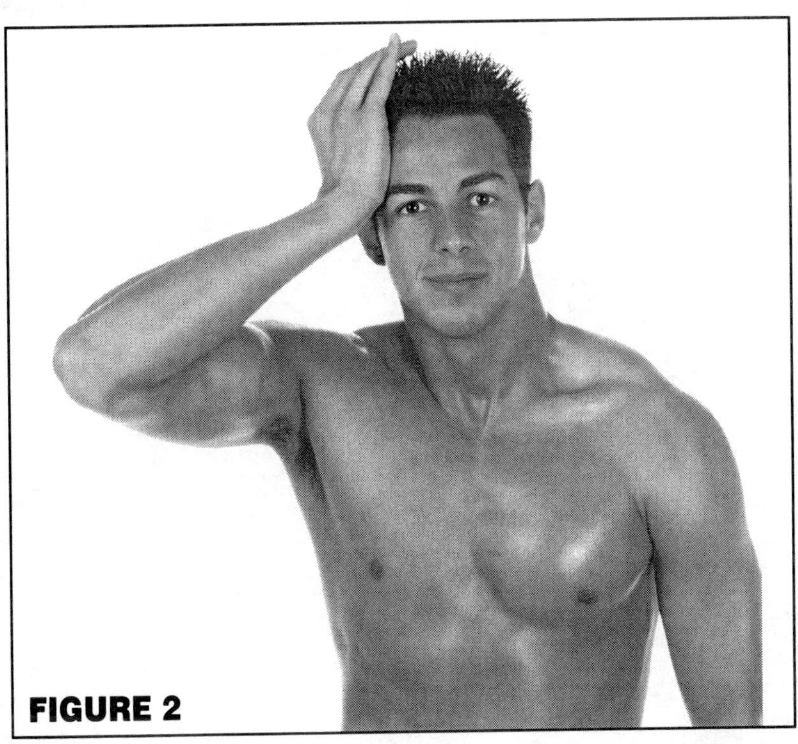
FIGURE 2

#5—GIRAFFE FLEX II

This PowerFlex® will give your neck a good stretch as you complete the workout. Sit or stand, facing forward. Bow your head to the right as far as you can without straining. Slowly roll your head, rotating your neck in clockwise circles. Reverse the movement and repeat, rotating your neck counter-clockwise.

There you go: five PowerFlexes to help you build a strong, well-muscled, attractive neck. These PowerFlexes aren't hard to do, but if you do them consistently and patiently, you'll help protect your neck from injury and enhance your bodies overall performance.

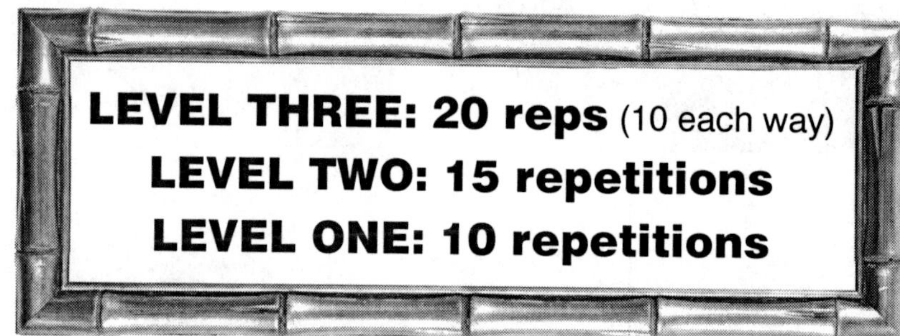

LEVEL THREE: 20 reps (10 each way)
LEVEL TWO: 15 repetitions
LEVEL ONE: 10 repetitions

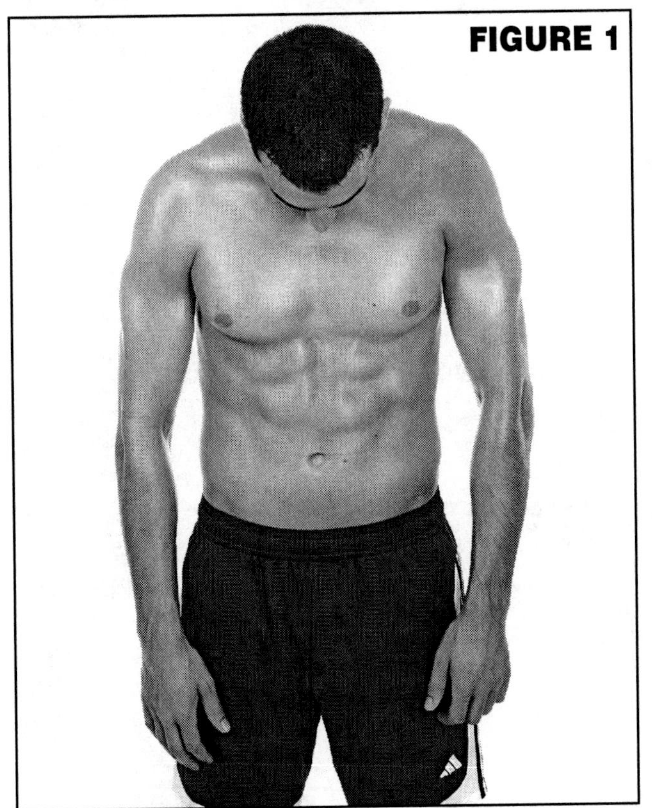
FIGURE 1

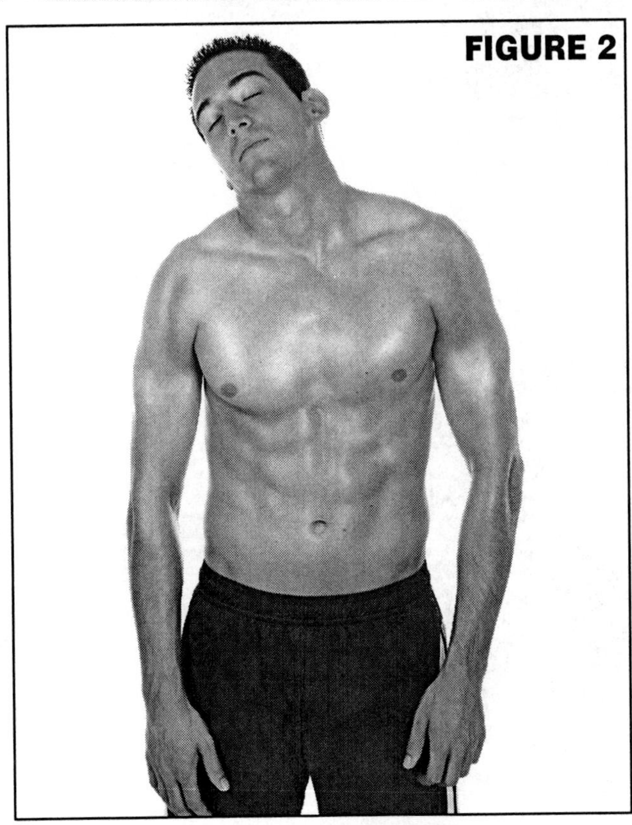
FIGURE 2

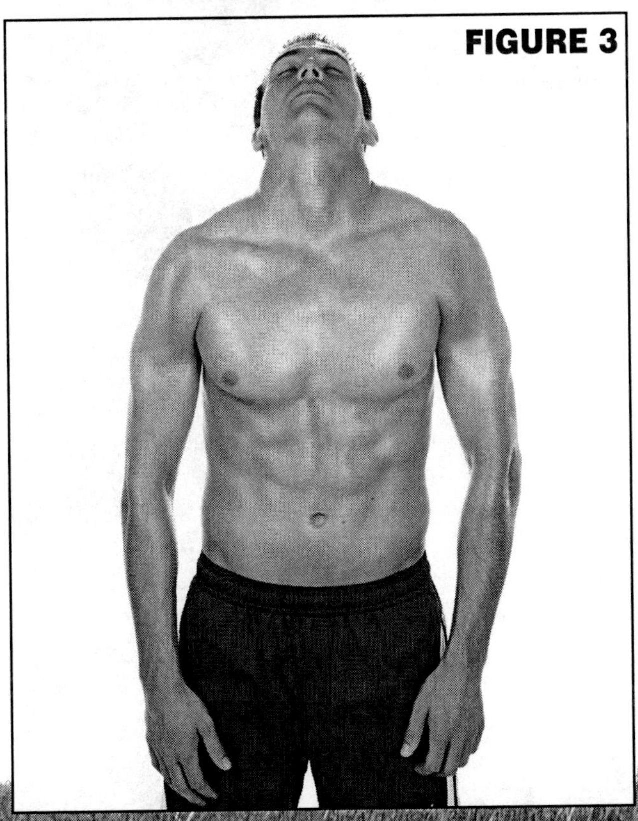
FIGURE 3

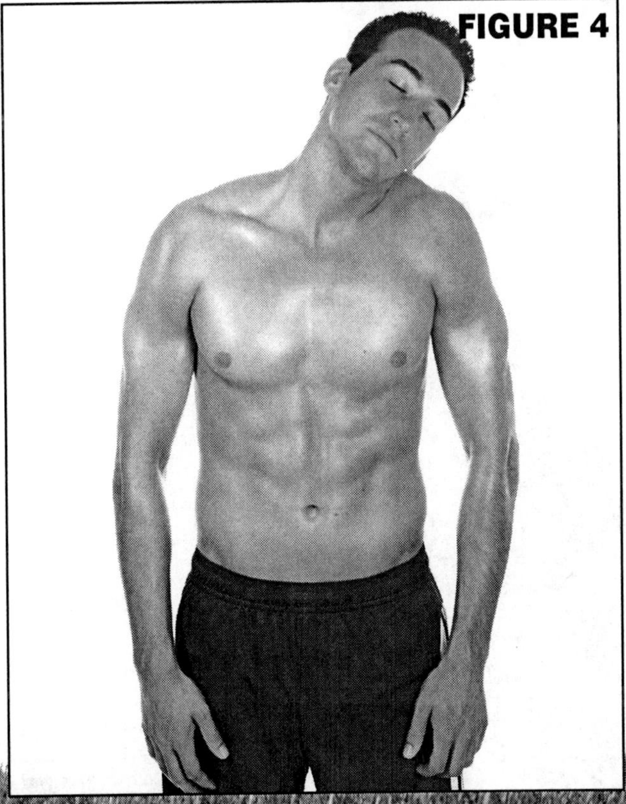
FIGURE 4

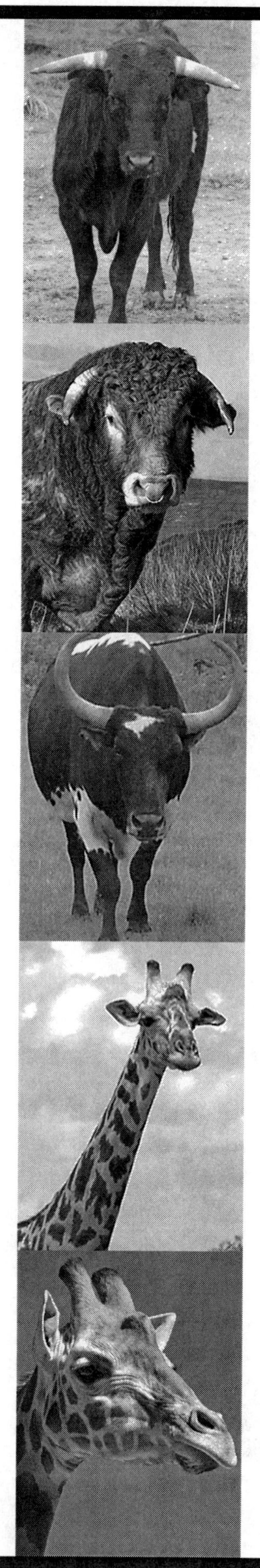

Neck Exercises

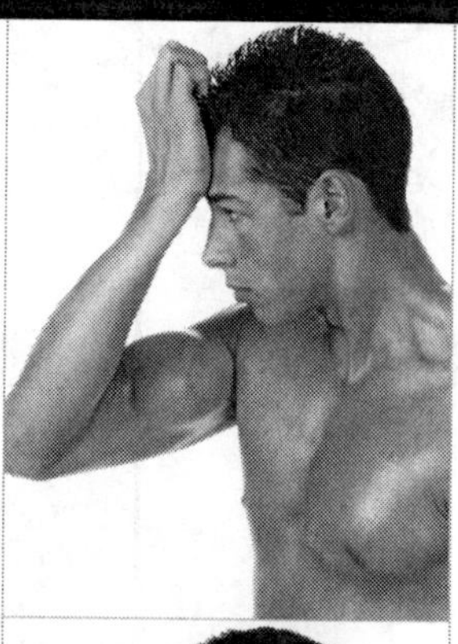

BULL FLEX I

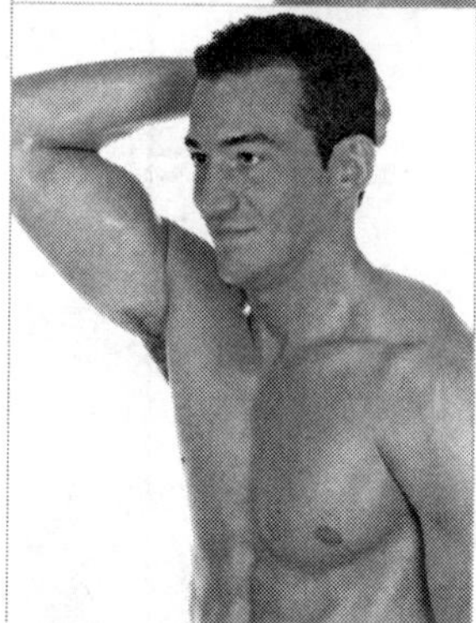

BULL FLEX II

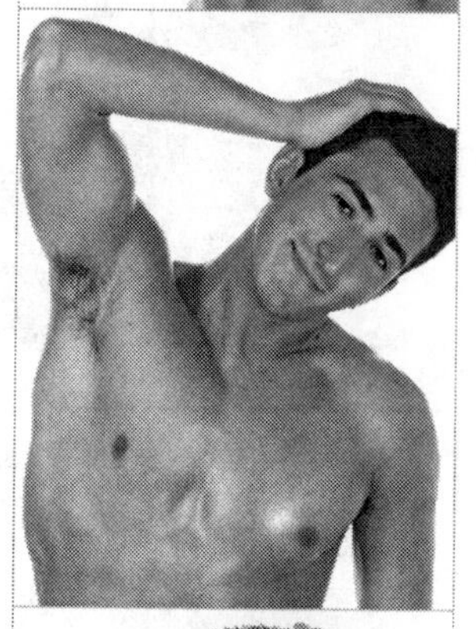

BULL FLEX III

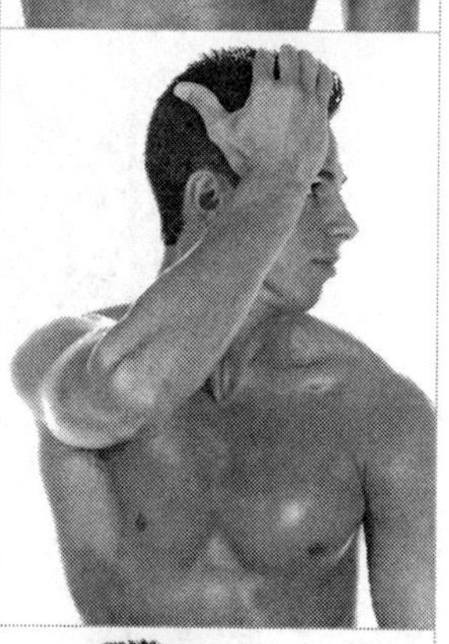

GIRAFFE FLEX I

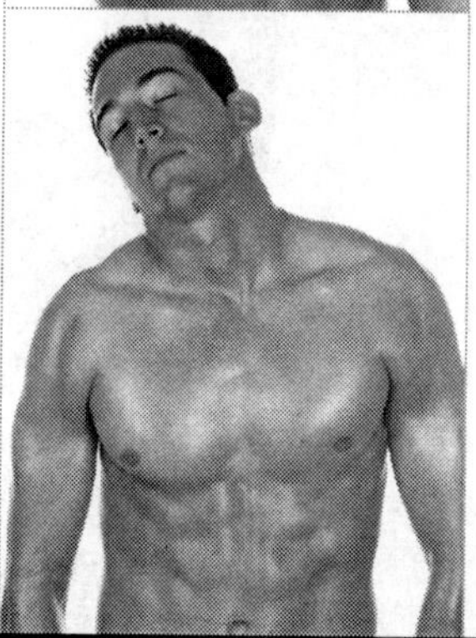

GIRAFFE FLEX II

POWERFLEX *Back*

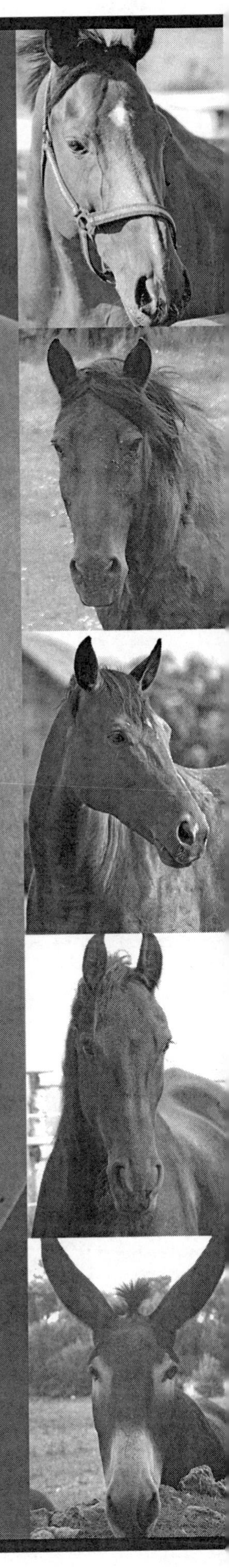

BACK WORKOUT

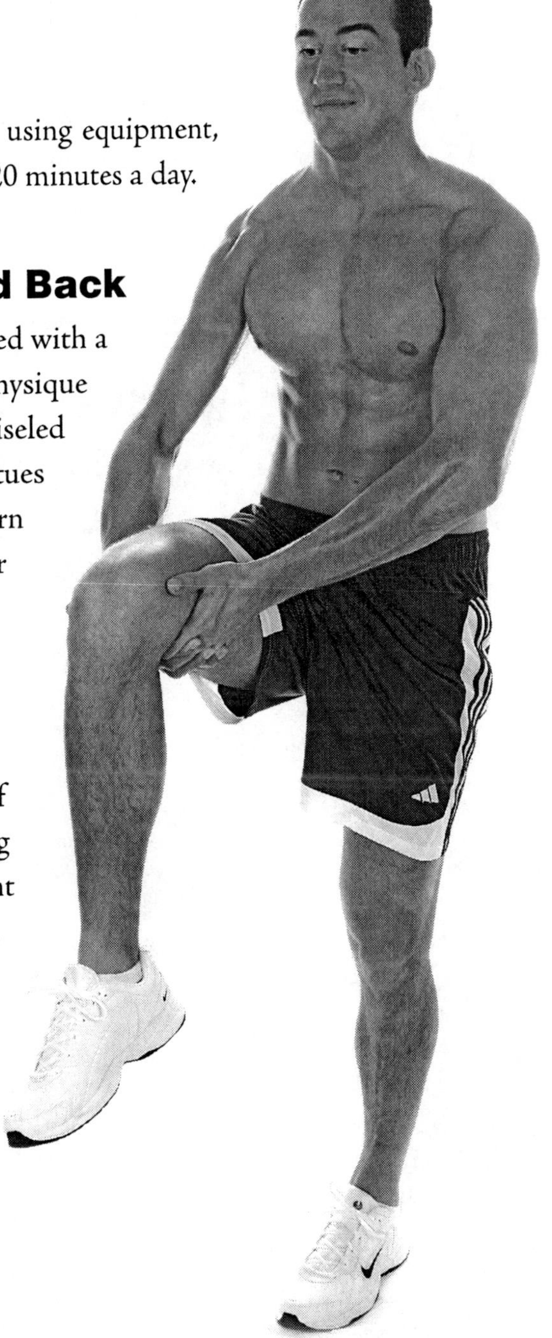

You can have a muscular, attractive, powerful back without using equipment, weights, pulleys, or machines. Just do five PowerFlexes for 20 minutes a day.

Wild Workout® for a Muscular, V-Shaped Back

A well developed chest with a flat rippling stomach combined with a healthy muscular back is something so attractive to the human physique that it has been the center theme of many artist of old, who chiseled their master pieces of the stone into works of art, priceless statues of the human form possessing these qualities of the body to adorn the palaces and halls of royalty. Yet when considering the power and beauty of a power muscular back none surpass the attraction and beauty which is possessed by the horse. When noticing the broad beauty and strength of the horses back, notice also it is associated with raw power to go with the good looks!

Its back has been carrying human riders since the dawn of time, along with packing supplies, carrying saddle bags, being strapped to wagons, carts, and even bearing the burden of a knight in shining armor lancet and all! Also, don't forget all modern day engines are rated to their horse power.

As you can see when it comes to a beautiful powerful muscular back the horse has the edge on the competition. Close behind though is also the pack mule which quite a bit resembles the horse. The movements of these precious animals will be simulated so you can have a beautiful powerful muscular back. Now let's get onto the Wild Workout® for a beautiful, muscular, powerful back!

#1—HORSE FLEX I

This PowerFlex® simulates the way horses' back muscles work as they pull heavy loads. It will help you improve your balance, too. Stand with your feet shoulder-width apart. Lean over and interlock your fingers behind your left knee, just above where it bends. Stand up slowly and smoothly, resisting with your left leg as you lift it. Do an equal number of repetitions as you resist with your right leg.

LEVEL THREE: 40 reps (20 per side)
LEVEL TWO: 20 repetitions
LEVEL ONE: 10 repetitions

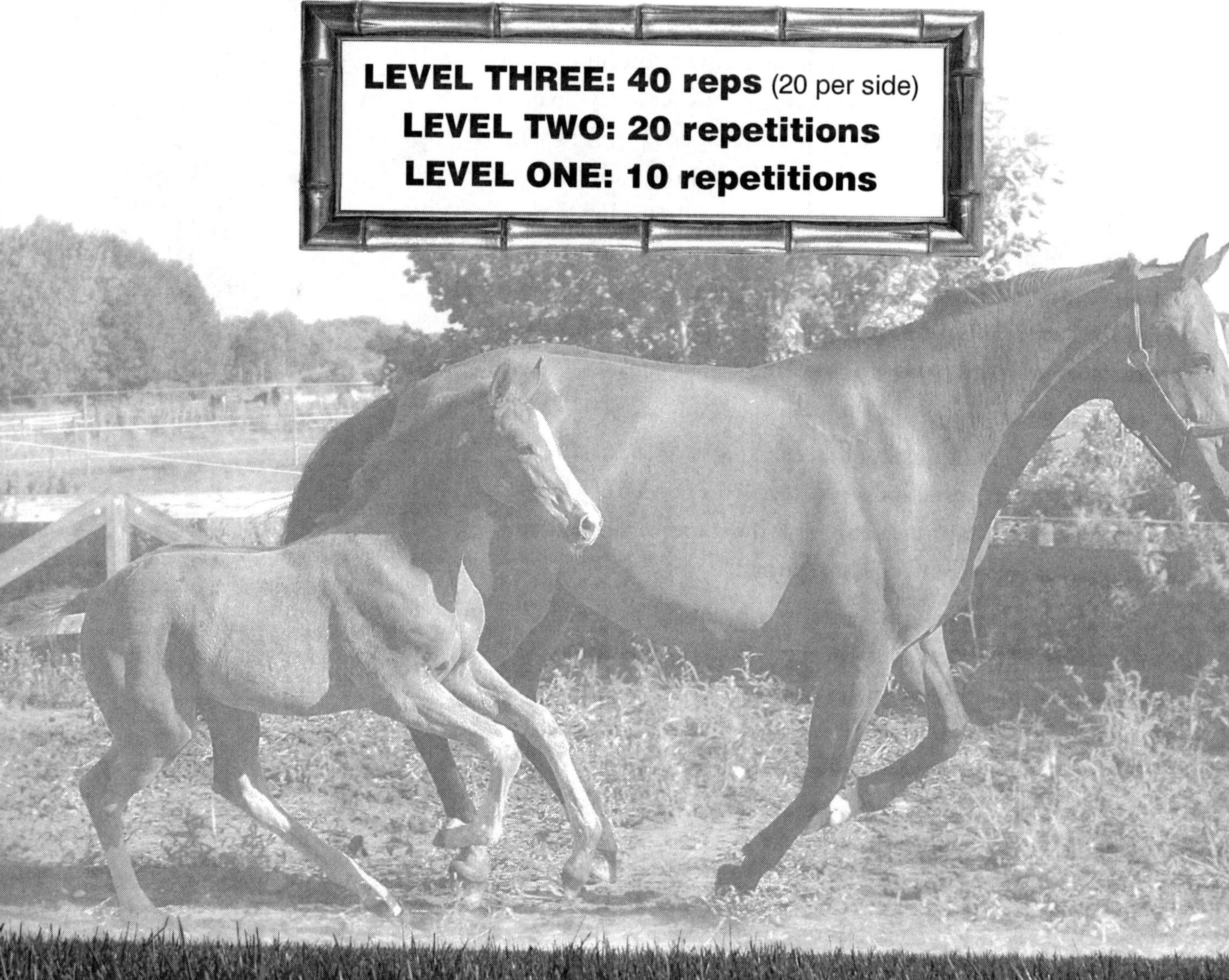

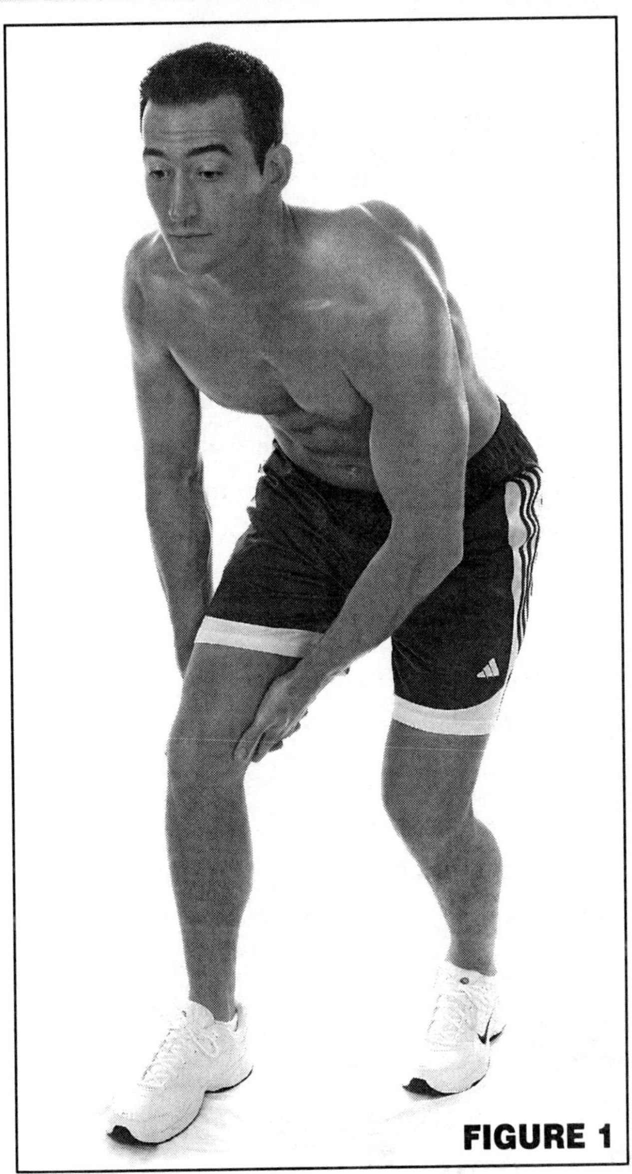
FIGURE 1

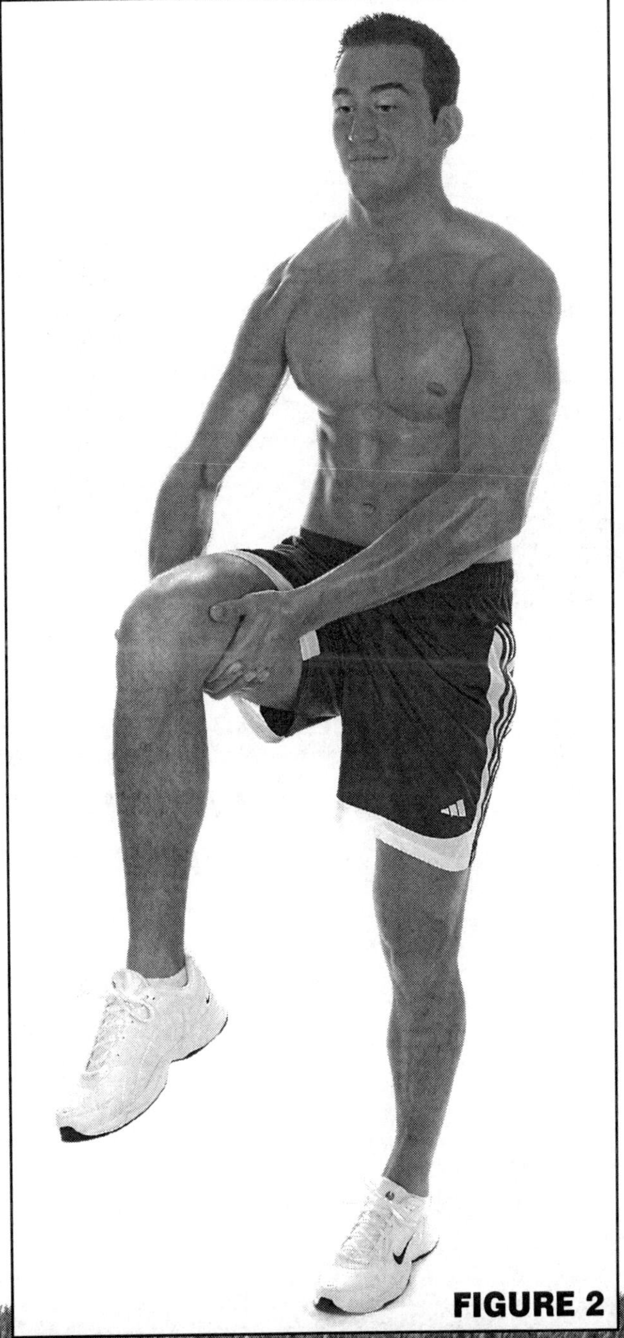
FIGURE 2

#2—HORSE FLEX II

To many fans, bucking bronco horses are the stars of the rodeo. "Broncs" explode out of the chute, their strong back muscles buck, flex, and whip upward with the force and power to throw a full grown rider for the ride of their life and toss them to the ground with a mouthful of dirt. This is the movement of the Horse Flex II. First, set a sturdy chair or stool a few feet away from a heavy piece of furniture, such as a bed, dresser, or couch (you may be able to use the same setup you used for Dolphin Flex III in the Abdominal Workout). Lay face down across the chair or stool and slide your feet under the bed, dresser, or couch. Place both hands behind your head, one atop the other. Slowly and smoothly, raise your upper body as far as possible. Then lower yourself.

It's okay if you can't raise your upper body very far at first. Do the best you can. With time, your strength and range of motion will increase. Just don't give up! This PowerFlex® is essential for building a strong, healthy, pain-free lower back.

You'll begin to feel the power of a strong back in no time at all, just keep at it. Never forget exercise is like bank account, you get out of it what you put into it and your body will thank you a million times over for continuing and not giving up. Stay at it! Remember all engines are rated according to their HORSE-POWER!

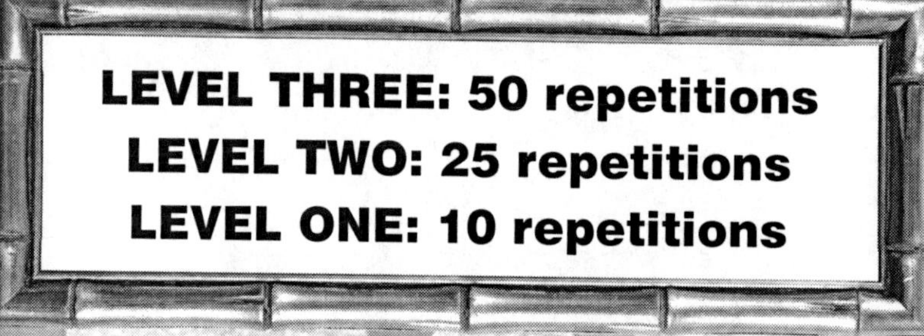

LEVEL THREE: 50 repetitions
LEVEL TWO: 25 repetitions
LEVEL ONE: 10 repetitions

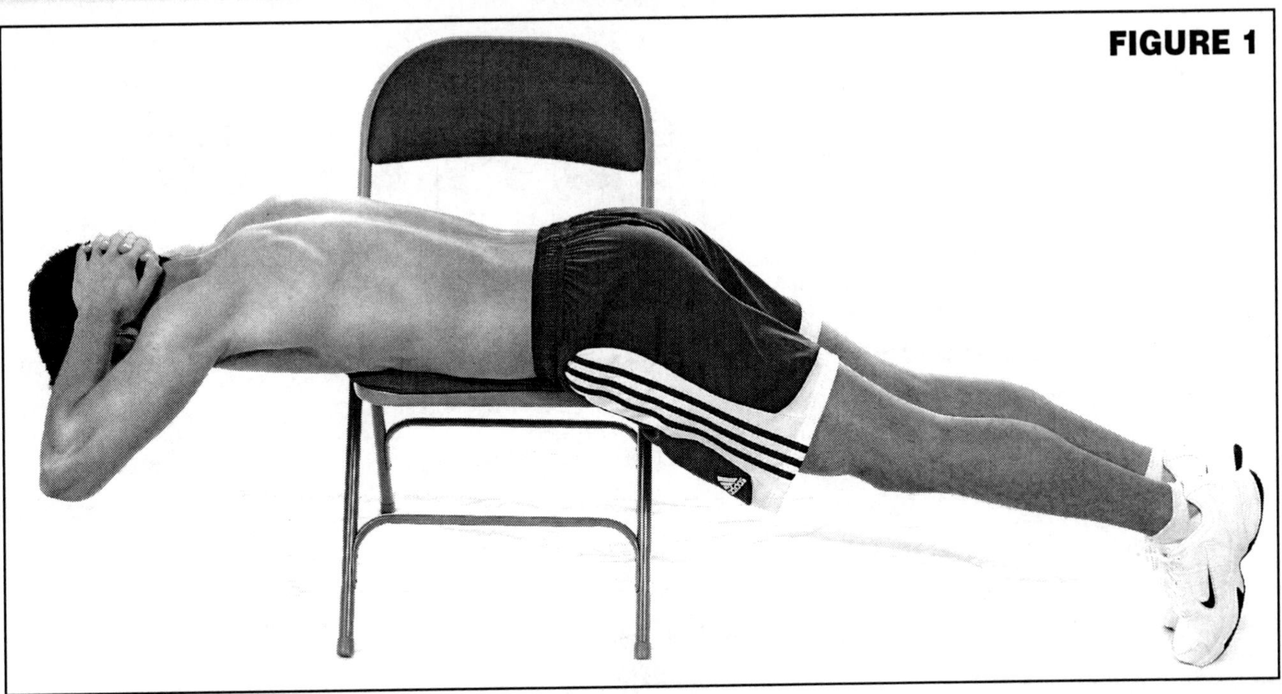

FIGURE 1

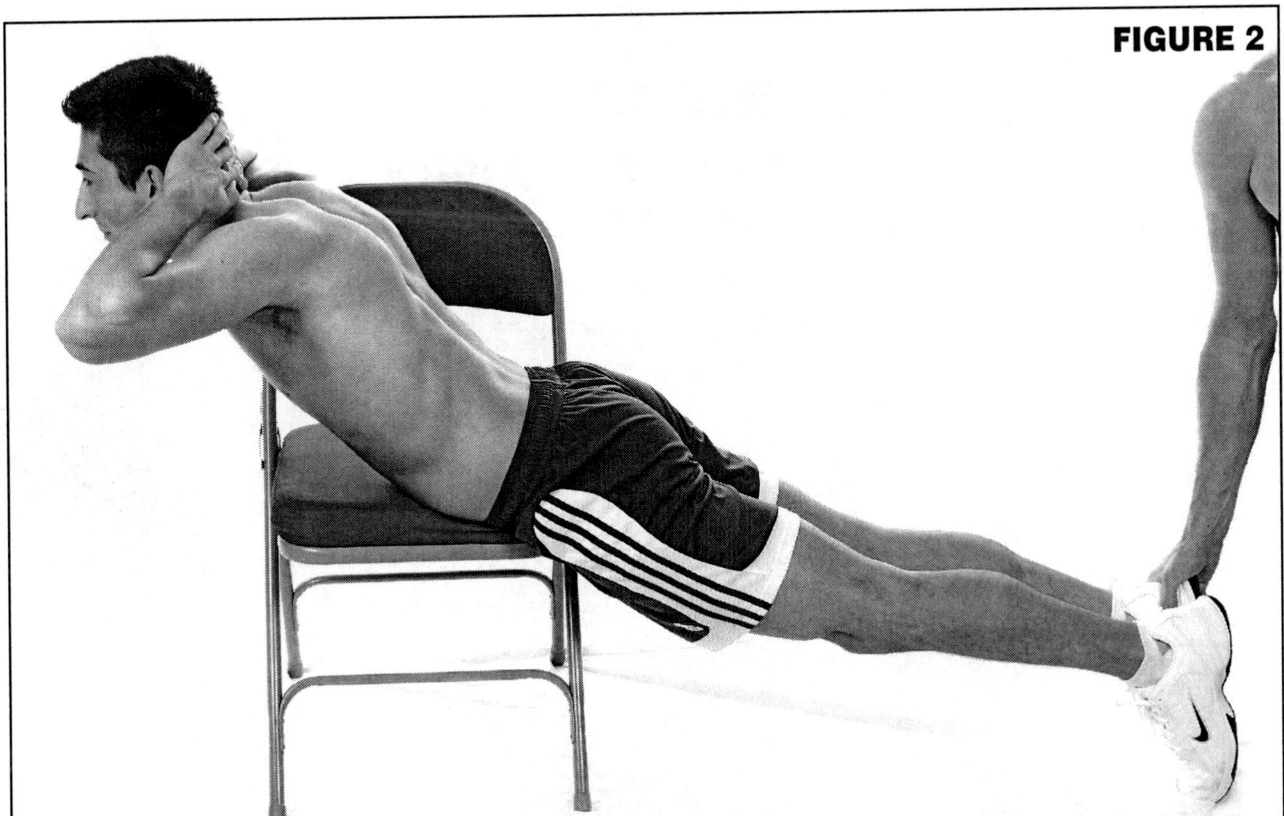

FIGURE 2

#3—HORSE FLEX III

Horses are undeniably graceful, from the way they run at the Kentucky Derby to their ability to flex and move their bulging back muscles in front of the saddle at will to shoo away flies. This PowerFlex® imitates that movement and works the upper back muscles.

Stand with your feet shoulder-width apart. Clasp your hands together behind your back at about waist height. Now push your shoulders back and down. Return to the starting position and repeat. Put a little extra effort into it and your muscles will really stand out. It may seem a little awkward at first, but do them with confidence and the movements will feel very natural after a short time. You will be amazed and pleased by the results—a strong, powerful, muscular back. Envision the goal of how you want to look while you are doing your PowerFlexes. It will help you put a little something into your workout and help you attain your goal. Keep at it. You can have the body you want. It is attainable. Just don't quit!

LEVEL THREE: 20 repetitions
LEVEL TWO: 10 repetitions
LEVEL ONE: 5 repetitions

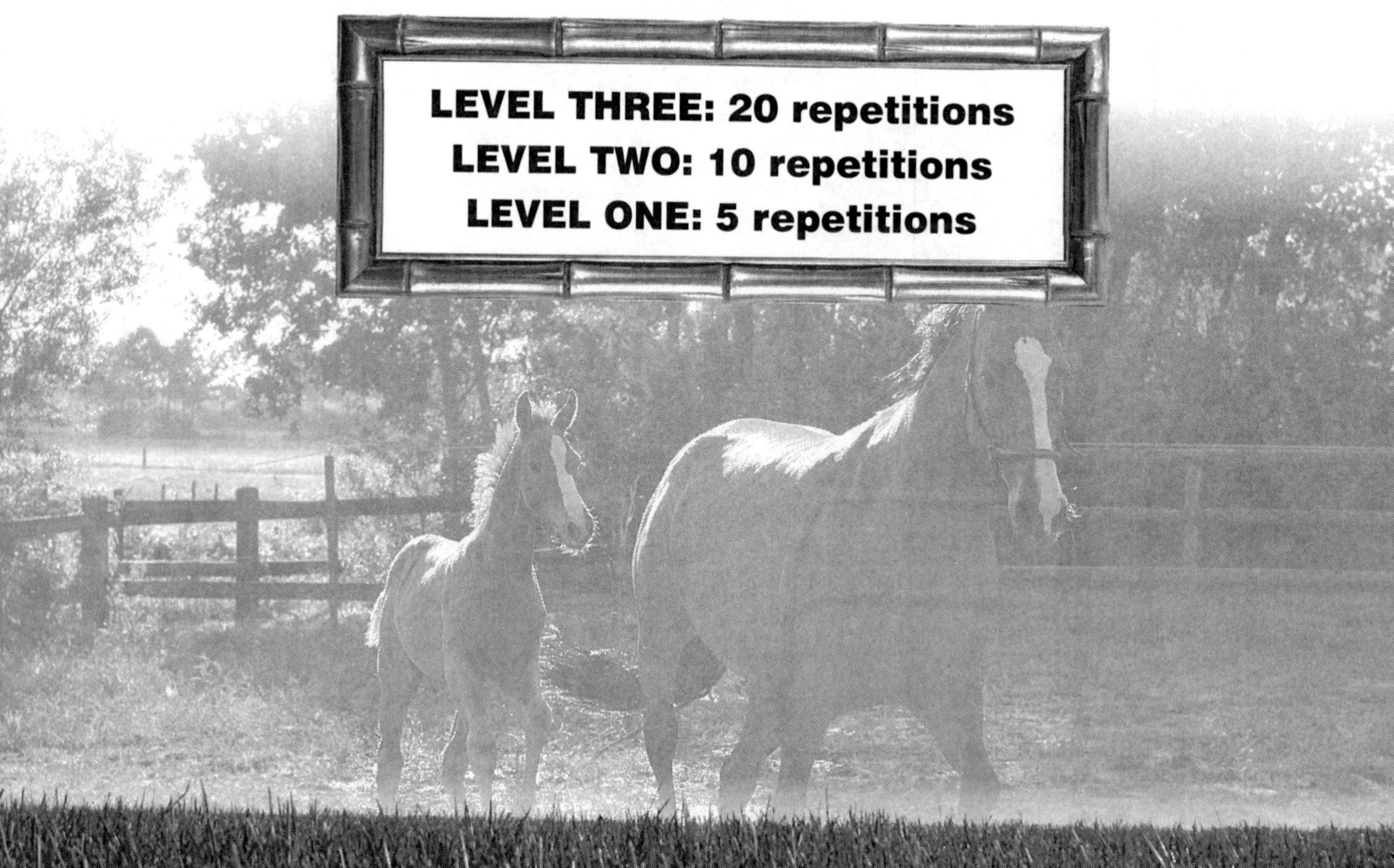

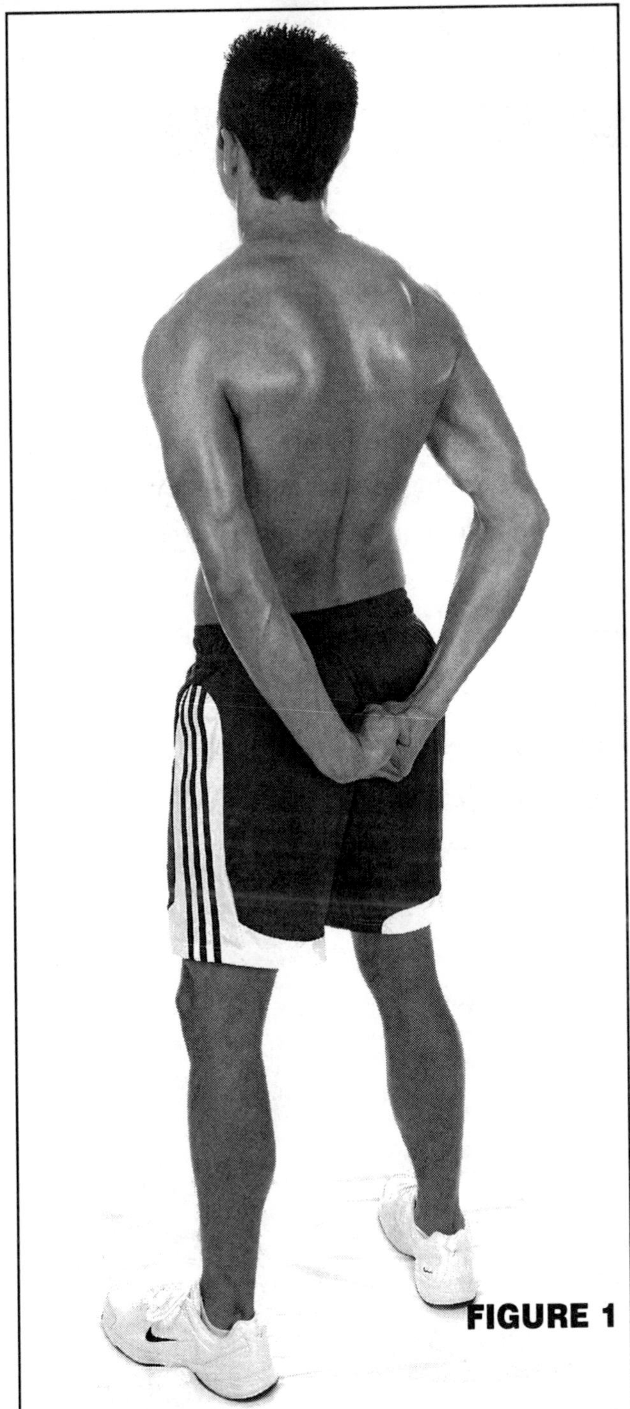
FIGURE 1

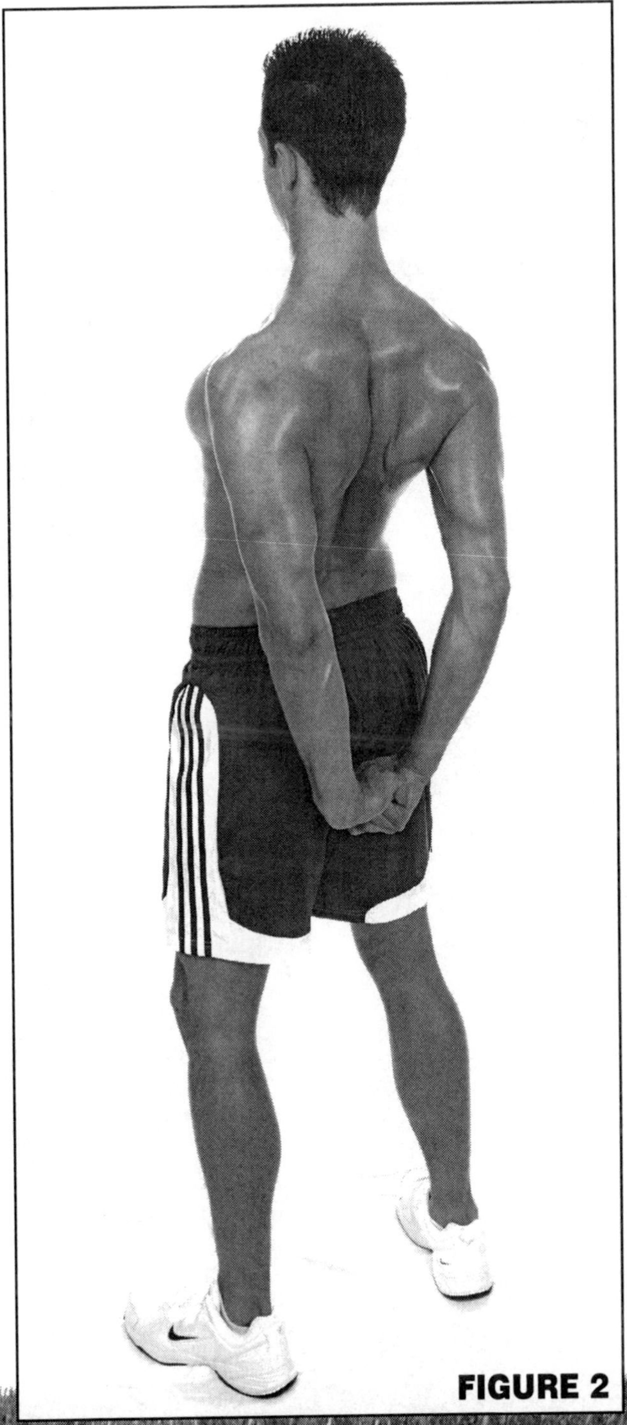
FIGURE 2

#4—HORSE FLEX IV

You'll look a little like a lucky horseshoe as you do this PowerFlex®. Practice it faithfully, however, and you won't need luck to keep your lower back strong and healthy.

Lie face down on a soft carpet or mat. Clasp your hands behind your back. Slowly and smoothly arch your back and, at the same time, raise your legs. Pause for a moment and feel your muscles tense. Lower your torso and legs and repeat. Similar to Horse Flex II, this one can be difficult at first. It takes practice to coordinate the movements, but keep at it. Your coordination will improve with your strength.

LEVEL THREE: 15 repetitions
LEVEL TWO: 10 repetitions
LEVEL ONE: 5 repetitions

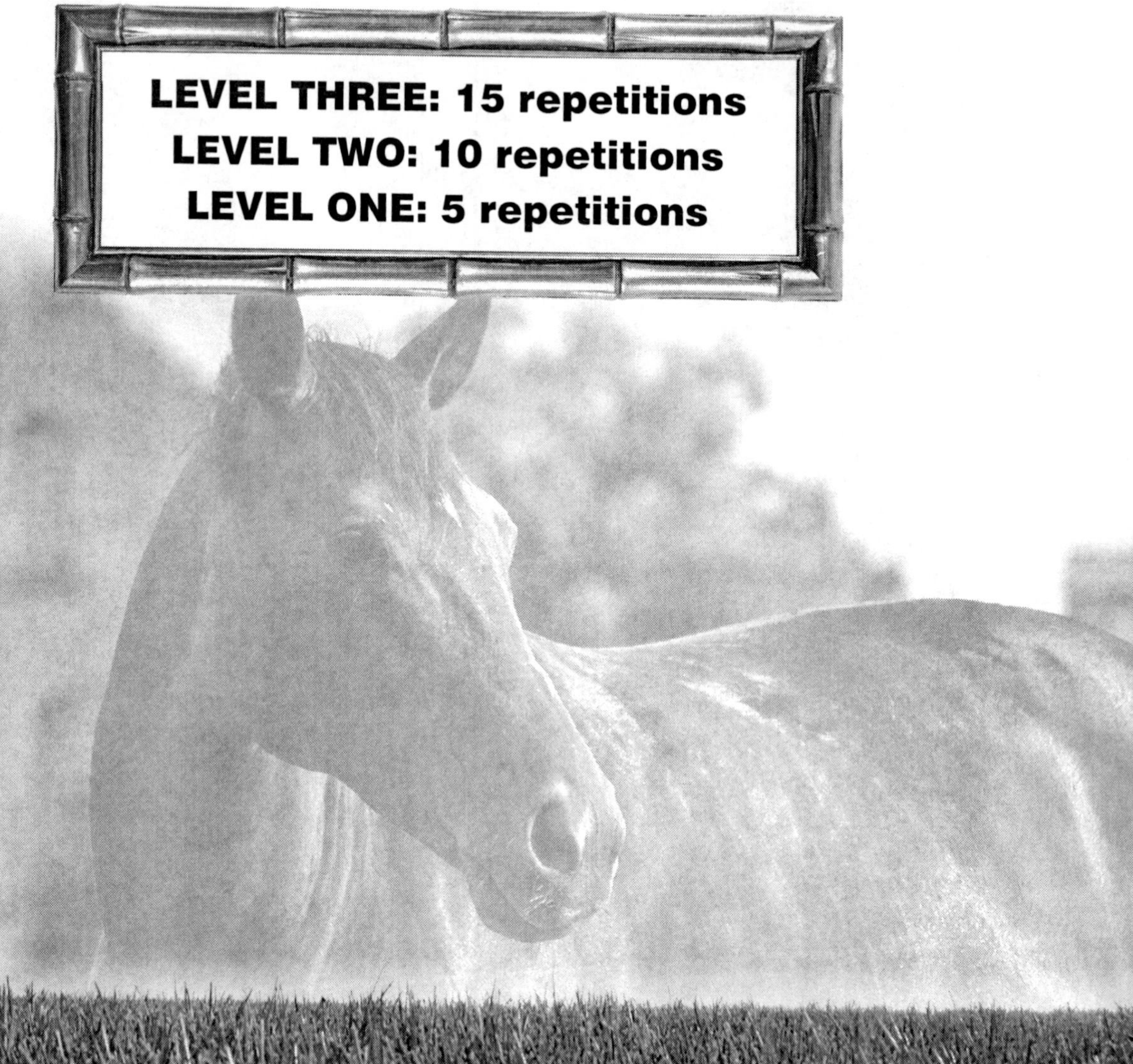

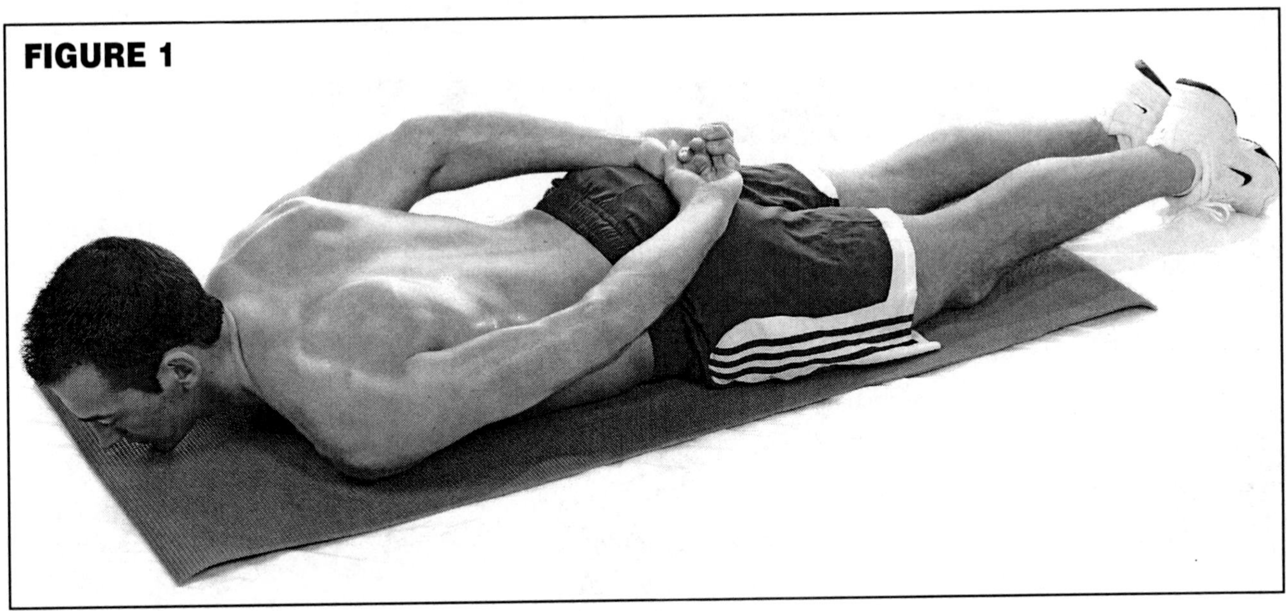

FIGURE 1

FIGURE 2

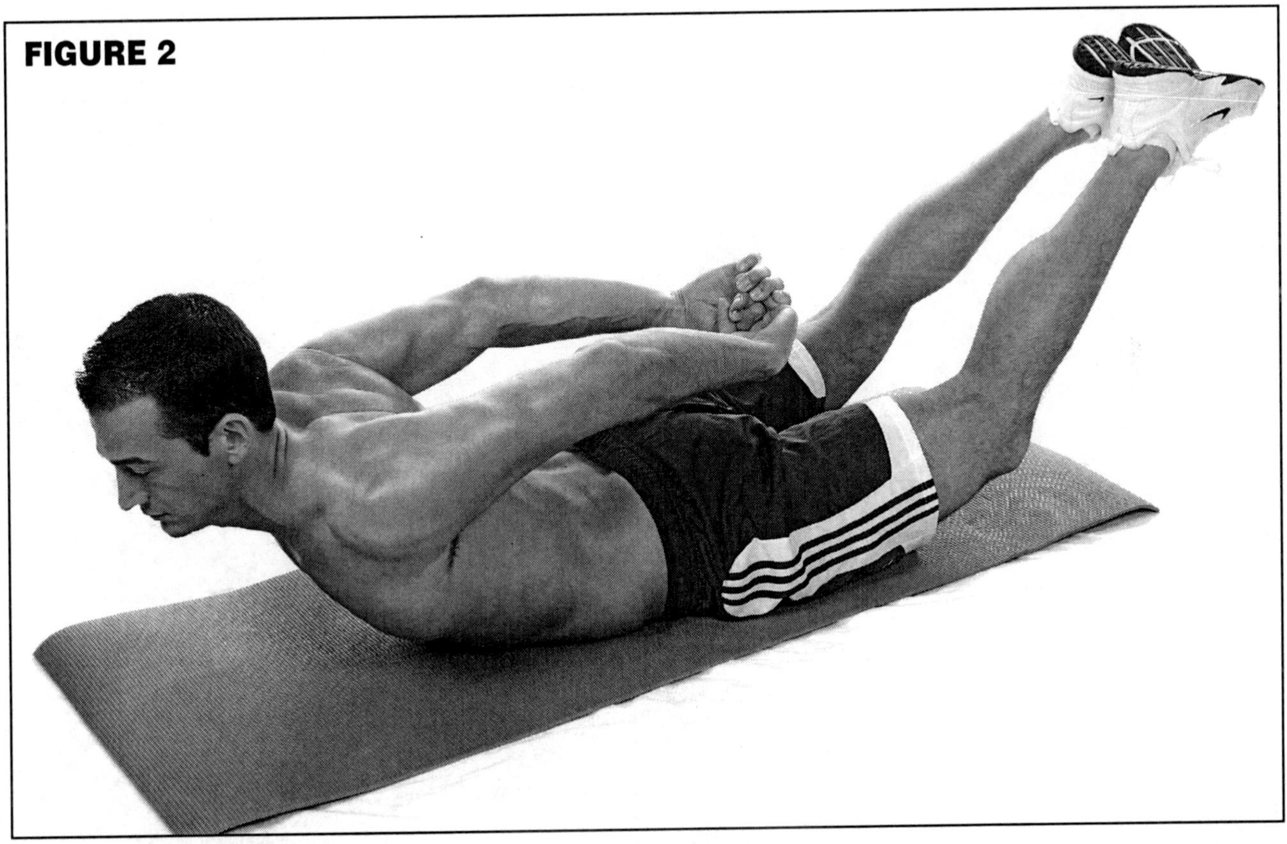

#5—MULE FLEX I

Unlike the horse, the mule isn't known for its grace but for the raw strength it uses to carry and pull immense loads that would break other creatures' backs. The last PowerFlex® in this workout imitates the way the mule bends and straightens itself beneath a load. Stand with your feet shoulder-width apart. Keeping your legs straight, reach to touch the floor, now smoothly stand back up and raise your hands above your head; not straight up above your head but each arm at a 45 degree angle like trying to touch where the ceiling and wall meet. Now slowly bend backwards and push your arms on to another like your trying to touch the top of your hands together while yet keeping your arms straight. Like a pack mule with a heavy load pushing down on the back just about pushing it down into the ground with legs sprawled straight out at the side. That's it you got it, now lower your arms and repeat.

There you go, friend. Practiced with consistency, determination, and patience, these five PowerFlexes will not only stretch and strengthen every muscle in your back but will teach your body to coordinate and use that strength.

So how does a person get the body they so desperately want? Work it out, continue, stay at it, put something into it, and keep working it out! The human body responds quickly! It is the only thing that gets better the more you use it. The Wild Workout® shows you how to use it to get the development you're looking for, it does work, get rid of the excuses, and get at it. Your body will say thank you, thank you, thank you, now get at it!

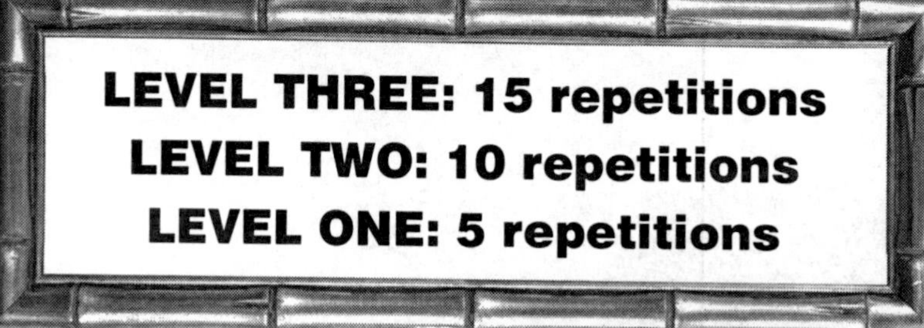

LEVEL THREE: 15 repetitions
LEVEL TWO: 10 repetitions
LEVEL ONE: 5 repetitions

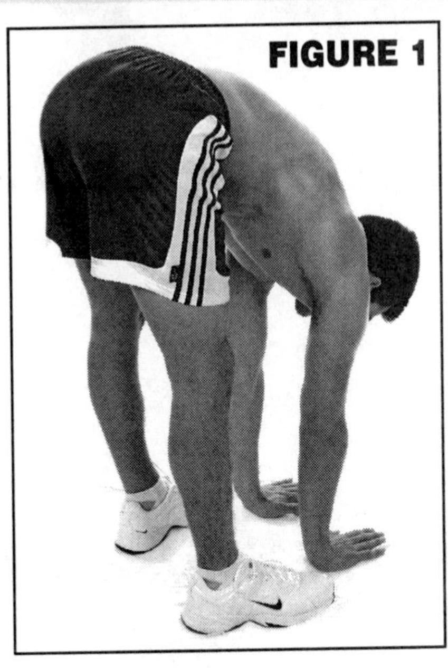

FIGURE 1

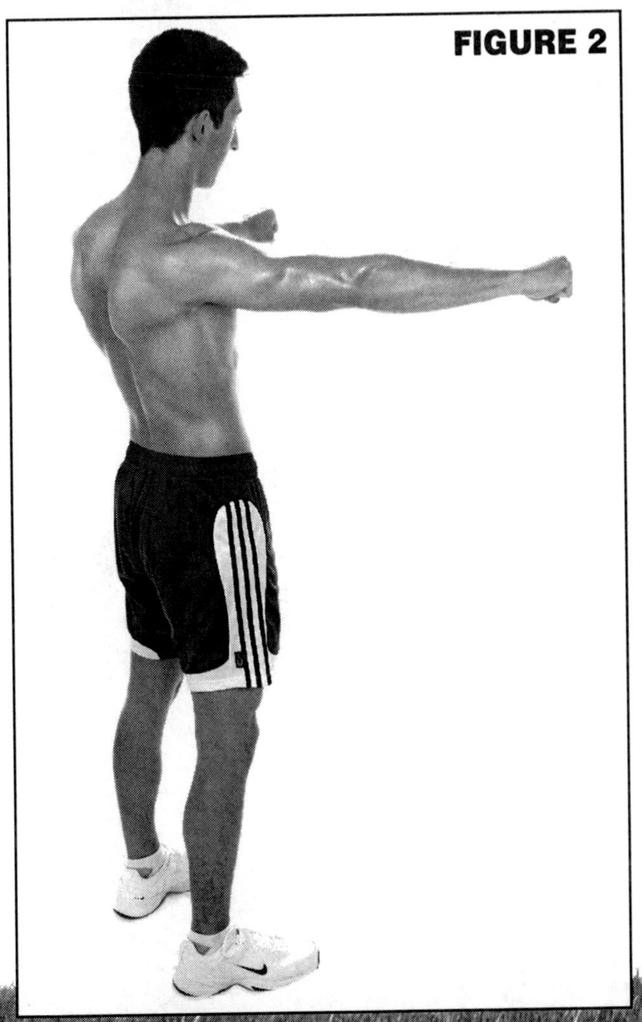

FIGURE 2

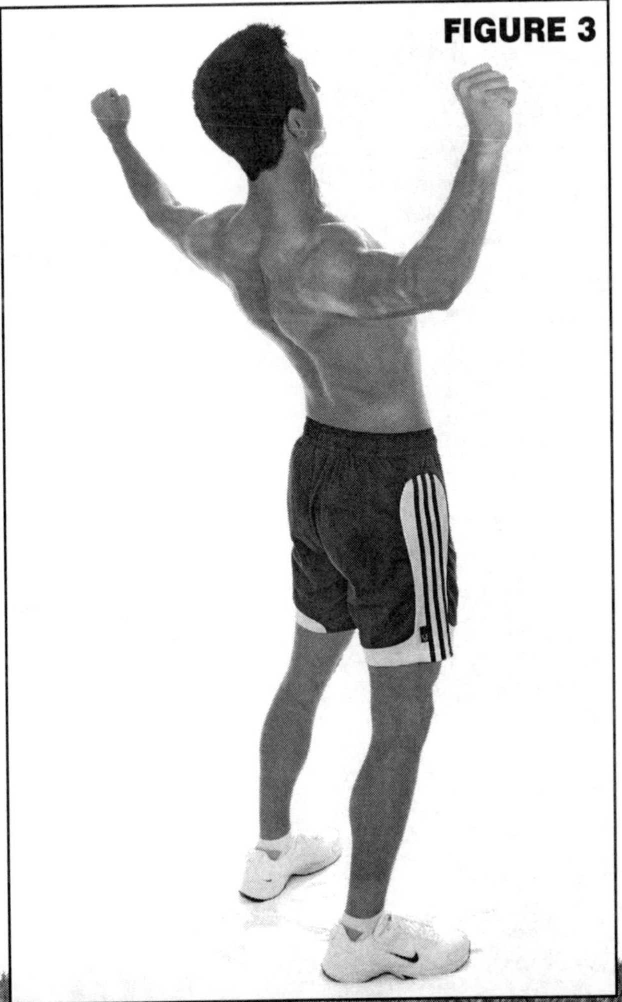

FIGURE 3

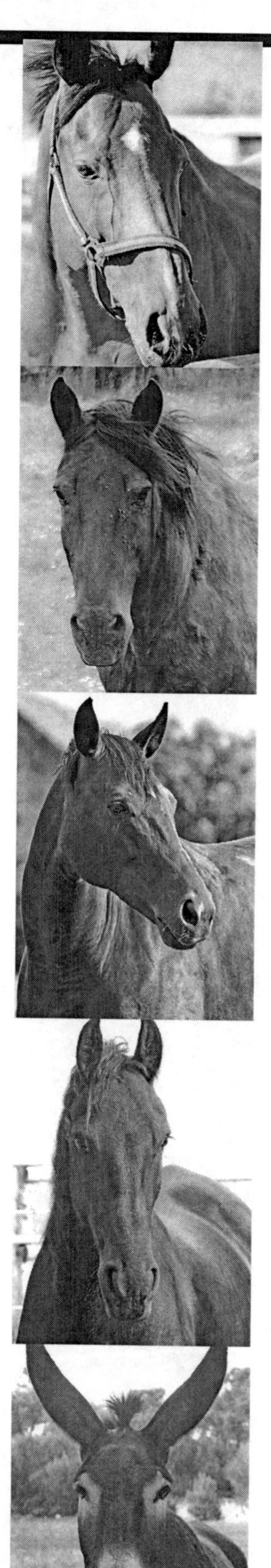

Back Exercises

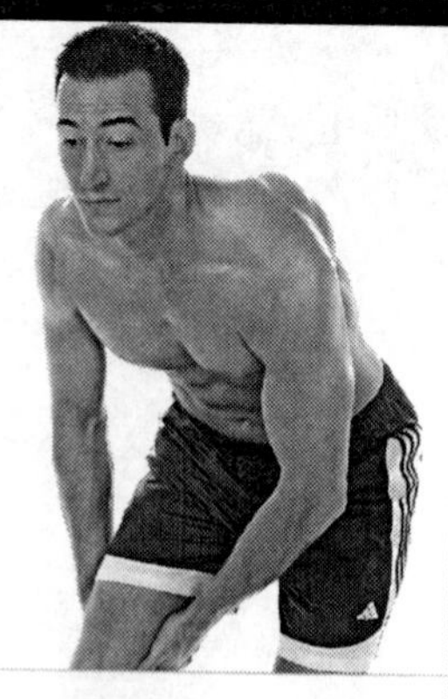

HORSE FLEX I

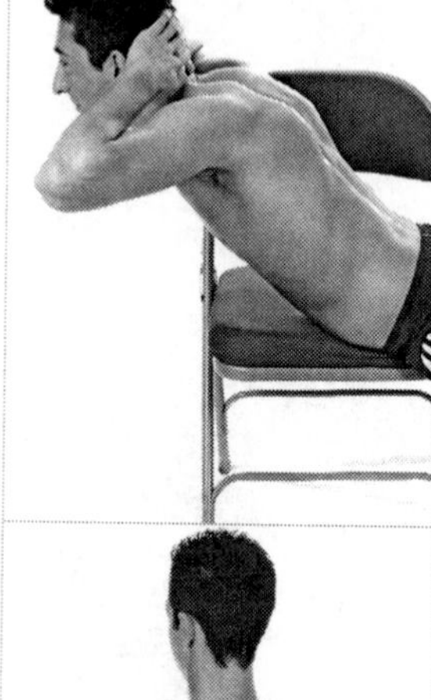

HORSE FLEX II

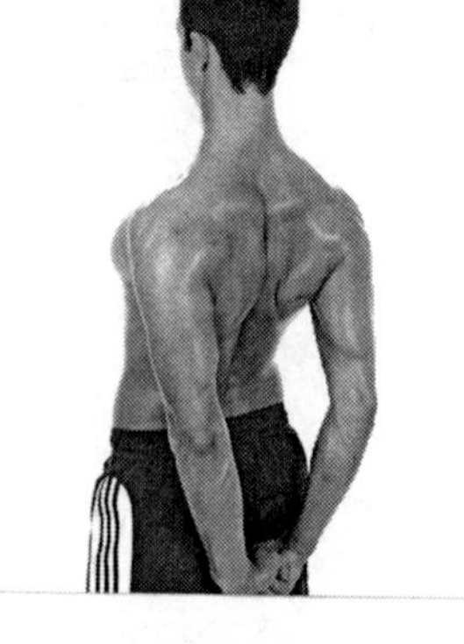

HORSE FLEX III

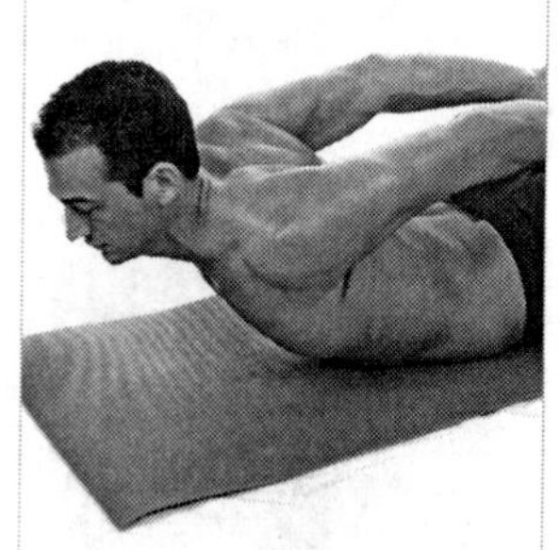

HORSE FLEX IV

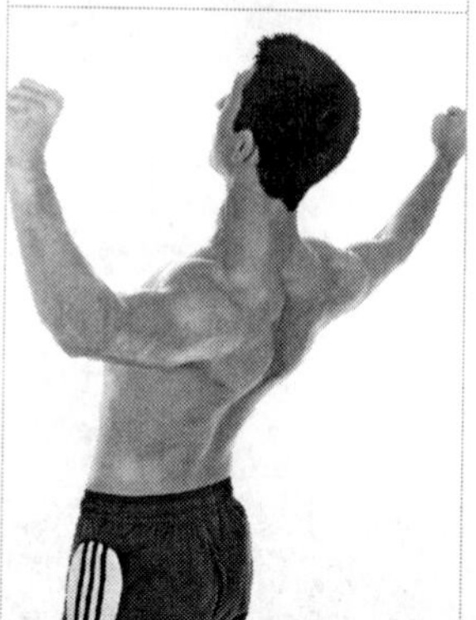

MULE FLEX I

HOW ARE YOU DOING?

Hey, wow, how many compliments have you gotten so far? How about that image you are seeing looking back in the mirror, pretty awesome huh! How about the difference you have noticed in your body's strength, flexibility, energy, the added bounce in your step, and feeling great! How about the difference in how your clothes are fitting; loose in the right places and tight where your muscles are developing! I commend you my friend but don't stop now-keep going! Yes, you can do it! Let me give you some inspiring words of encouragement—Never forget, a priceless diamond is just a lump of coal that just stuck with it. You my friend are starting to sparkle, your body is beginning to shape, your muscles are beginning to sculpt, your physique is beginning to define, and you are becoming a diamond harder than tempered steal, so keep at it my friend you are doing great!

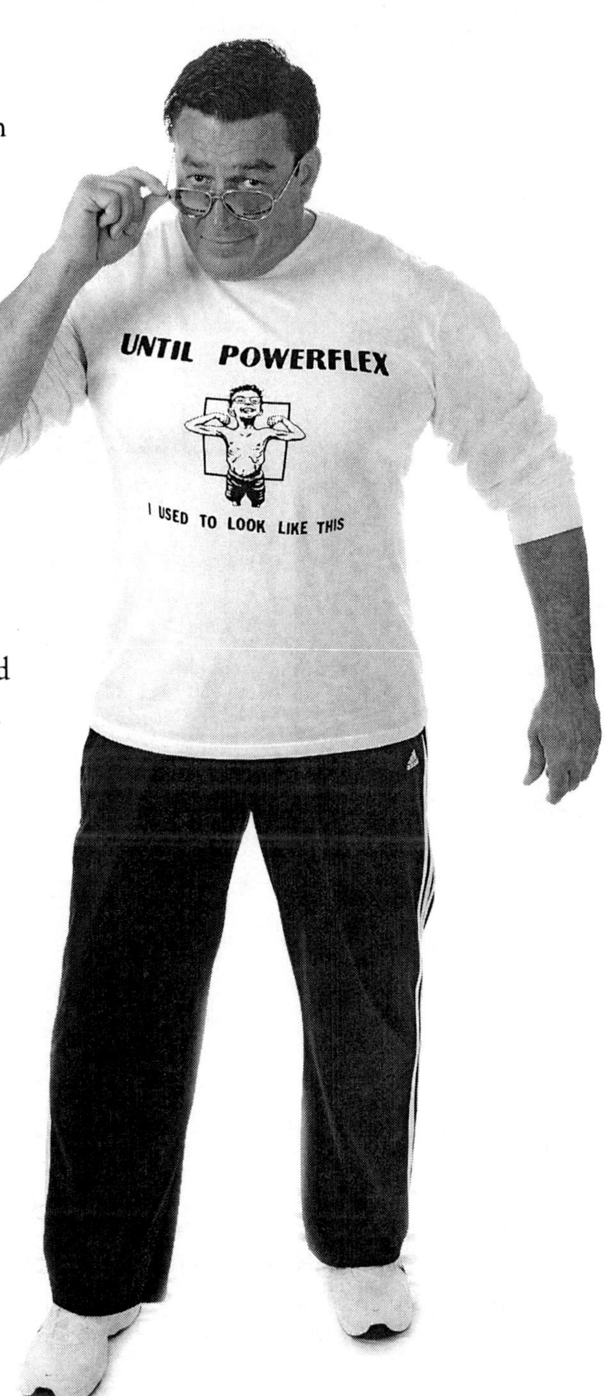

Sincerely,

The Forystek's

Creators of the Wild Workout®

DON'T QUIT

When things go wrong, as they sometimes will,
When the road you're trudging seems all uphill,
When the funds are low, and the debts are high,
And you want to smile, but you have to sigh,
When care is pressing you down a bit,
Rest if you must, but never quit.

Life is strange, with its twists and turns,
As everyone of us sometimes learns,
And many a failure turns about
When he might have won, had he stuck it out.
Don't give up, though the pace seems slow:
You may succeed with another blow.

Success is a failure turned inside out,
The silver lining in the cloud of doubt.
And you can never tell how close you are.
It may be nearer, when it seems so far.
So stick to the fight when you're the hardest hit.
It's when things seem worst that you must not quit.

POWERFLEX *Legs*

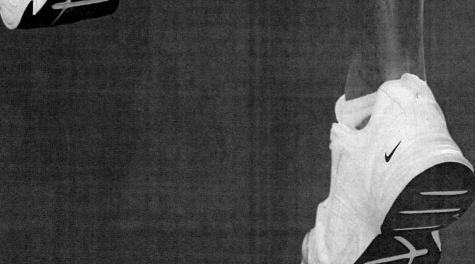

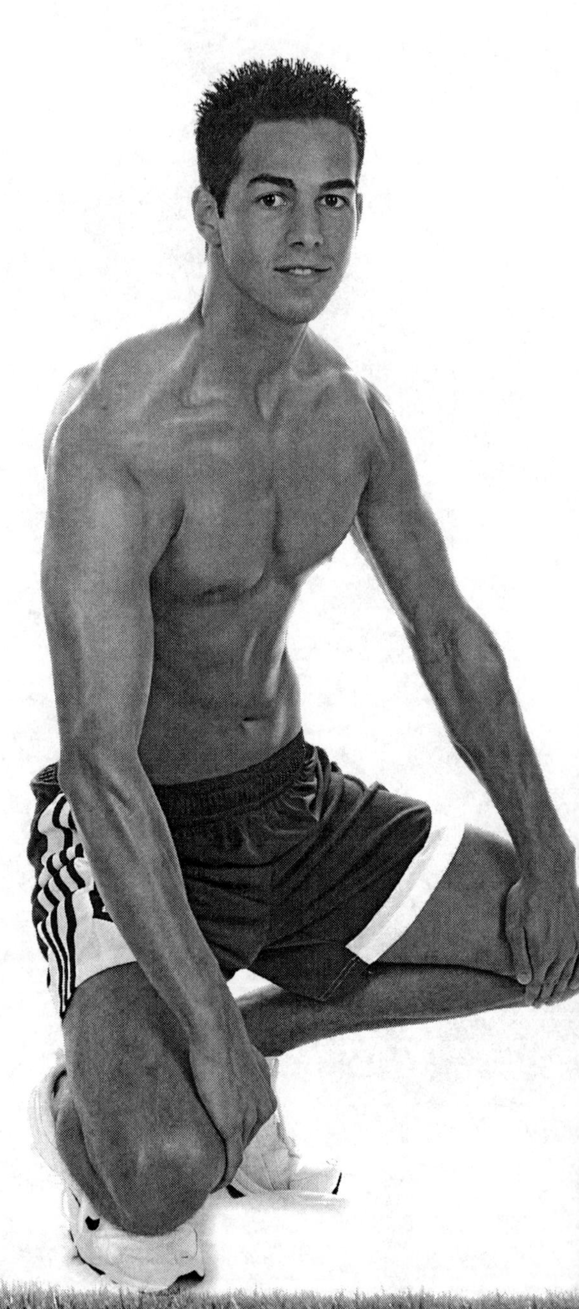

LEGS WORKOUT

You can have powerful, strong, attractive, muscular legs without using equipment, weights, pulleys, or machines. Just do five PowerFlexes for 20 minutes a day.

Wild Workout® for Powerful, Strong, Attractive, Explosively Athletic Legs

The legs play a great role in having a powerful attractive body. The legs carry the load of the rest of the body, so to have strong legs, with shape and muscles combined with power, does so much for the all around good of the entire body that its importance cannot be over emphasized

A good set of legs has not only been the center of many head turns and whistles but members of both sexes, but it is a powerful set of legs that has made the difference between winning and losing in many different forms of competition. The athlete that possesses powerful, strong, good-looking, muscular legs has the edge they need to come out on top.

There is one creature whose legs are known worldwide for their blast of power, strength, and amazing ability! As a matter of fact their legs are so desirable that in many parts of the world their legs are considered a delicacy and only the legs of this creature are eaten. There are national events centered totally around the amazing blast of power and strength processed by this creatures legs. This amazing creature is the frog! Its legs with the power to blast them in a leap many times longer than their body length has promoted this amazing creature above many animals bigger in size and ferocious in attitude, and it is the frog that has claimed the title for strong powerful legs, that can leap farther than its competitors! Its legs also possess great strength in swimming, so much so that it has inspired militaries around the world to slip on flipper (frog feet) and call their underwater divers frog men!

When it comes to strong healthy legs another vary unique animal comes into view, the kangaroo. This amazing creature can travel great distances even when carrying riders in its pouch by jumping and hopping on its powerful, strong legs! It seems like a big fluffy, lovable, harmless creature but don't be fooled, this creature has such leg power that one of its main defenses is to kick its attacker with such raw power that one blow from its powerful legs can end an intruders life instantly; human or animal. The kangaroo leans back on its thick tail freeing up its legs to be weapons! It has the legs, the power, the strength, the muscularity and it knows it!

The Wild Workout® for powerful strong, attractive, muscular legs is based on the principal of the amazing frog and kangaroo. Now let's get WILD!

#1—FROG FLEX I

For this PowerFlex® you'll imitate the frog's position as it springs off the ground— but without becoming airborne yourself. Stand with your heels close together and your toes pointing outward, forming a V. Place your hands on your hips and rise onto the balls of your feet. Keeping your back straight, bend your knees and lower your body as far as you can comfortably. Stay on the balls of your feet. Stand up again slowly and smoothly and repeat.

Balance can be tricky with this one. If you can't keep your hands on your hips and lower yourself without keeling over, it's okay to hold on to the back of a chair as you learn. As your confidence and strength improve, you'll find you won't need the chair. This PowerFlex® not only works your legs completely but also improves your balance.

LEVEL THREE: 100 repetitions
LEVEL TWO: 50 repetitions
LEVEL ONE: 25 repetitions

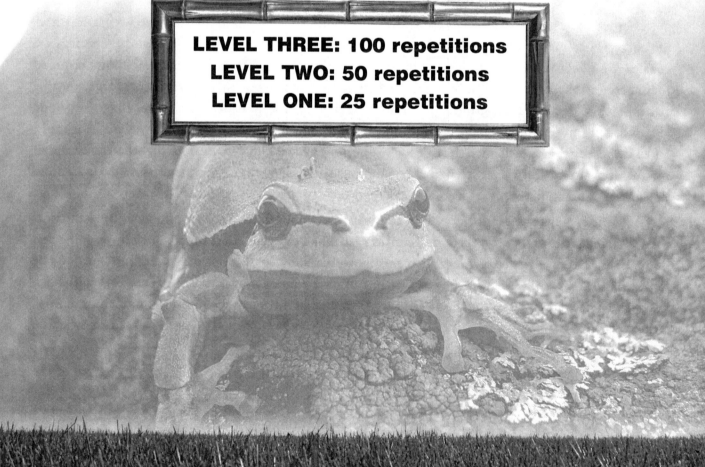

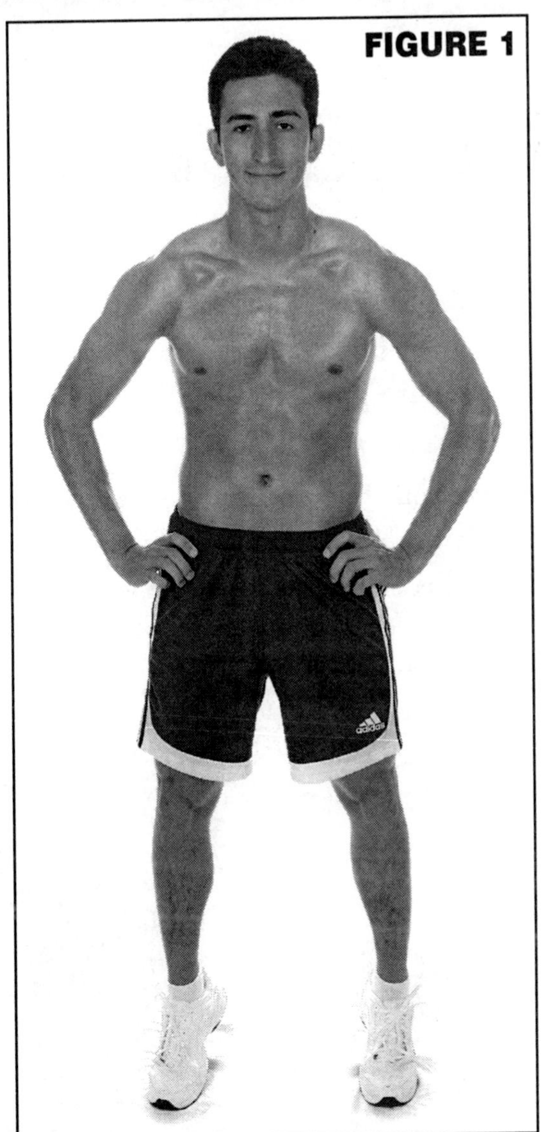
FIGURE 1

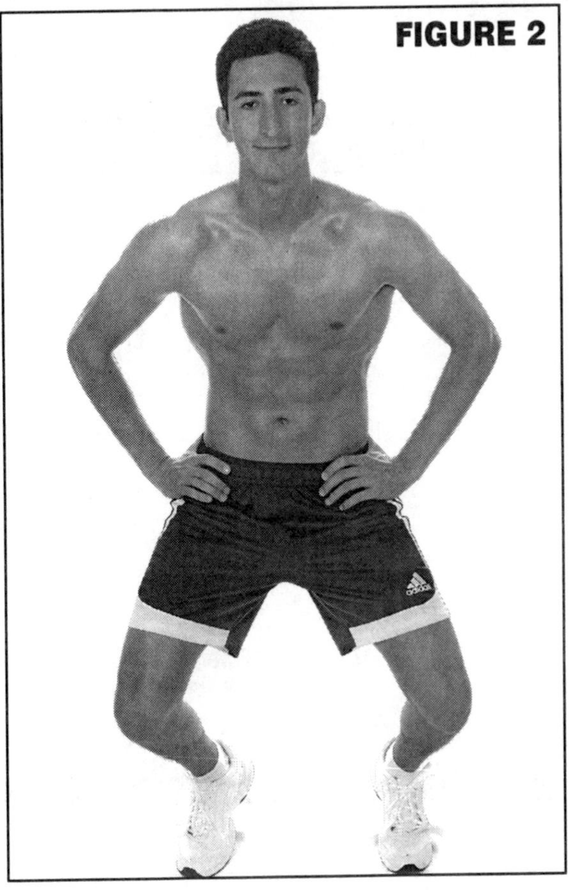
FIGURE 2

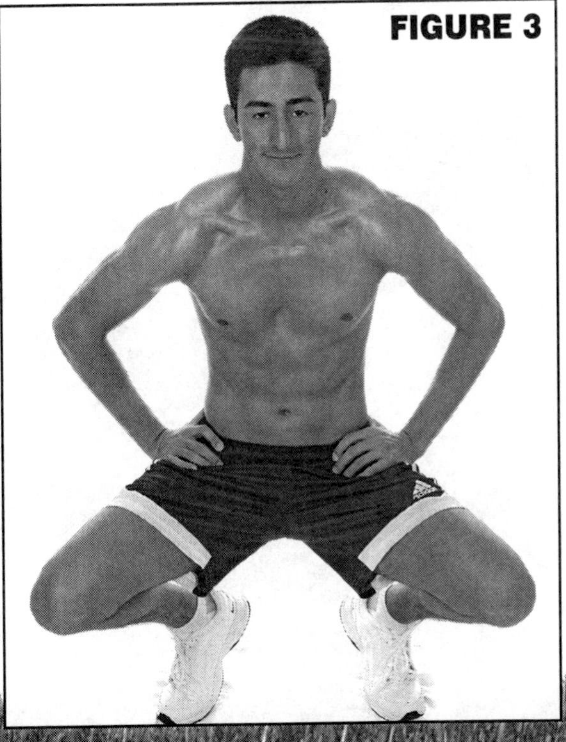
FIGURE 3

#2—FROG FLEX II

Here's a two-part PowerFlex® for the inner and outer thighs. First, squat down as far as you can comfortably—as though you're playing leapfrog— with your knees spread wide apart. Place the palms of your hands on the inside of your knees. Now try to push your knees together while resisting with your hands. Push and resist for a second or two, then relax and repeat.

For Part Two, squat down with your knees together. Place your palms on the outside of your knees. Try to push your knees apart while resisting with your hands. Push and resist for a second or two, then relax and repeat. Be sure to apply enough resistance to make this PowerFlex® challenging.

LEVEL THREE: 40 reps (20 per part)
LEVEL TWO: 20 repetitions
LEVEL ONE: 10 repetitions

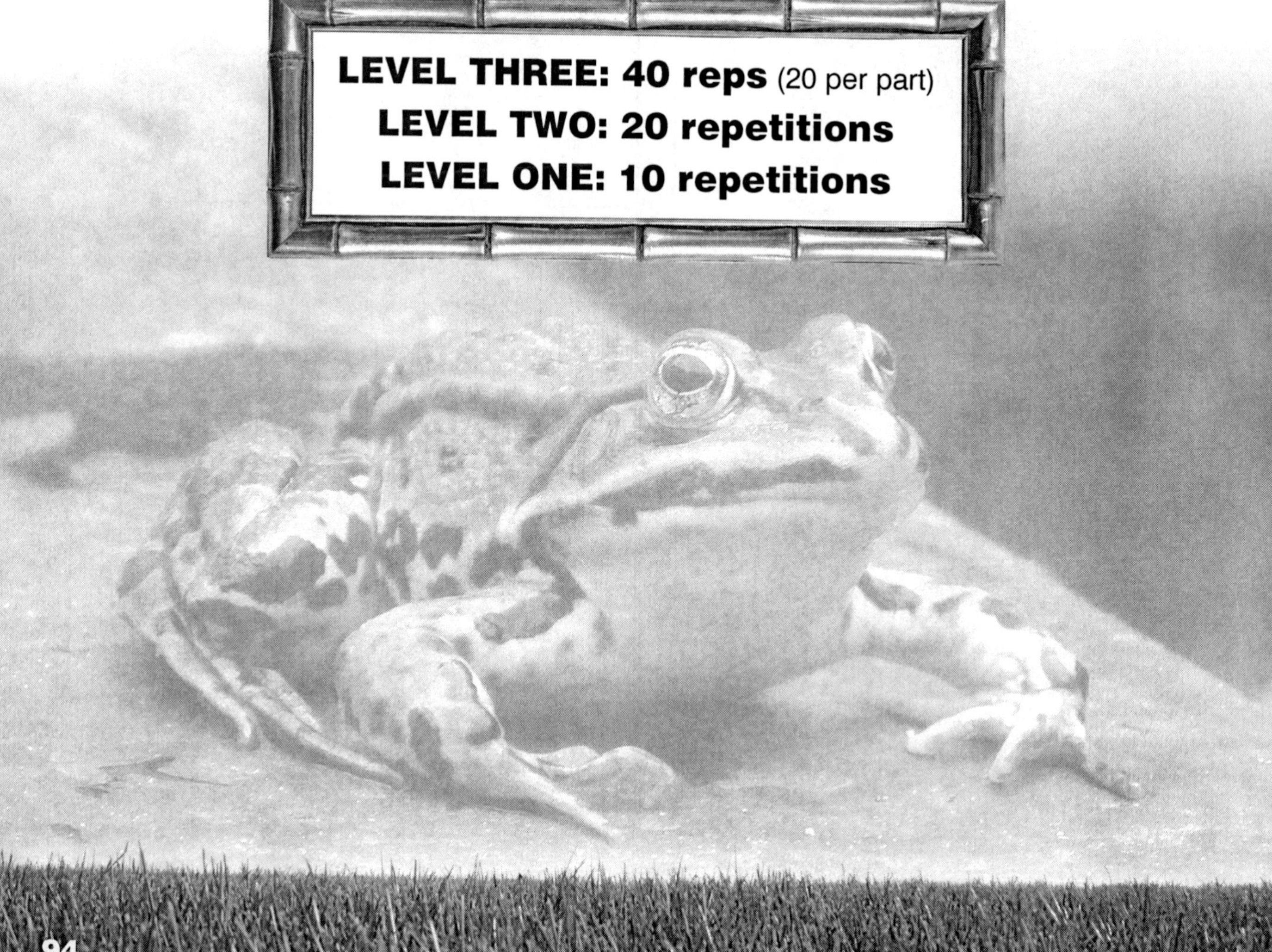

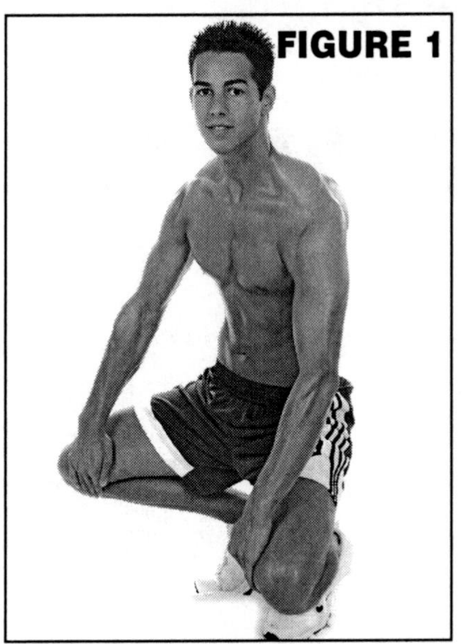
FIGURE 1

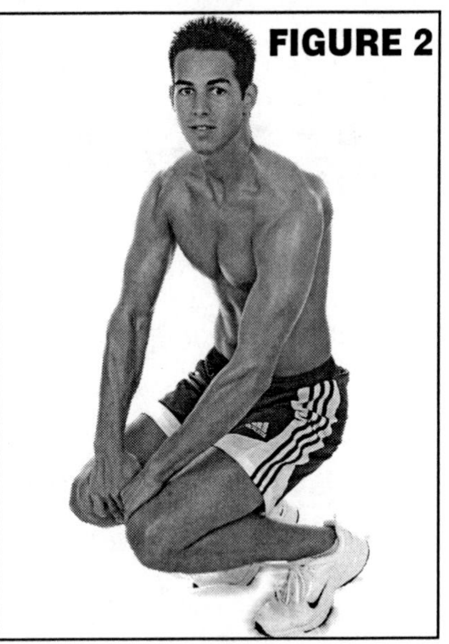
FIGURE 2

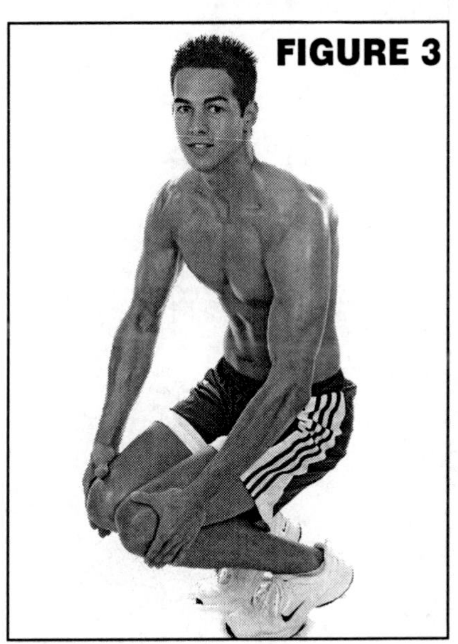
FIGURE 3

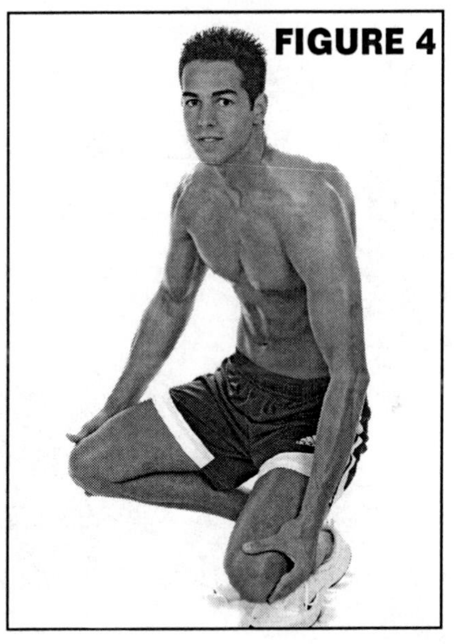
FIGURE 4

Modified

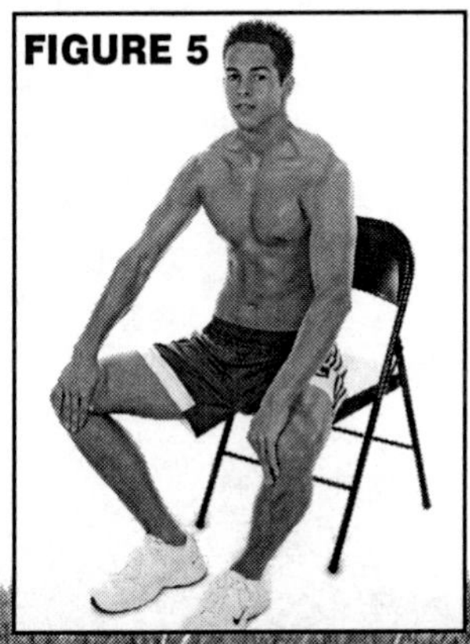
FIGURE 5

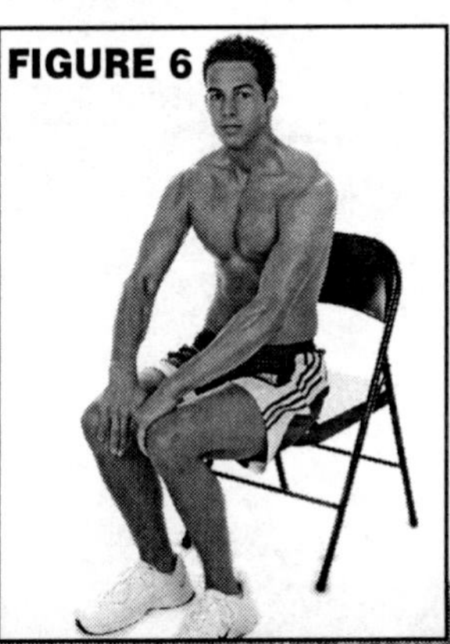
FIGURE 6

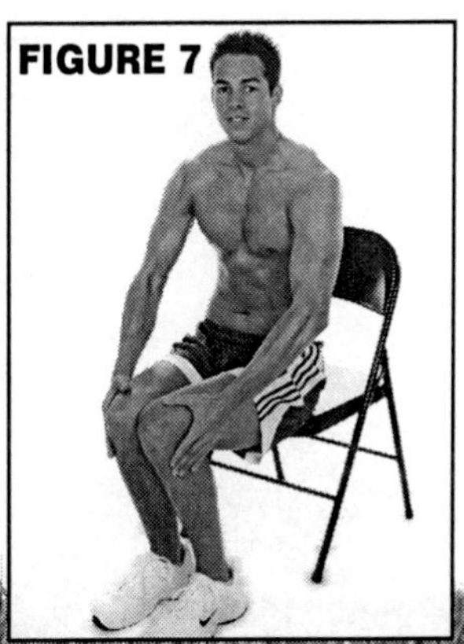
FIGURE 7

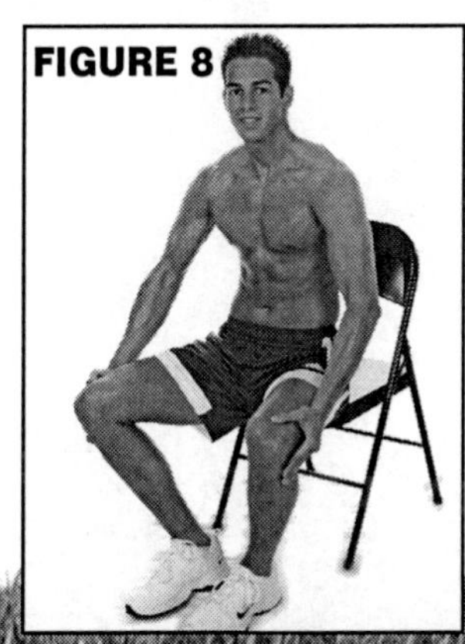
FIGURE 8

#3—KANGAROO FLEX I

This PowerFlex® simulates the kangaroo's position as it jumps, as Frog Flex I does the frog's. While standing, cross your legs (like a scissors), distributing your weight evenly on both feet. Hold your arms straight out in front of you. With your back straight, bend your knees and slowly lower your body as far as you can comfortably. Stand up again slowly and smoothly and repeat. If holding your arms in front of you doesn't help you keep your balance, it's okay to hold on to the back of a chair as you learn this PowerFlex®.

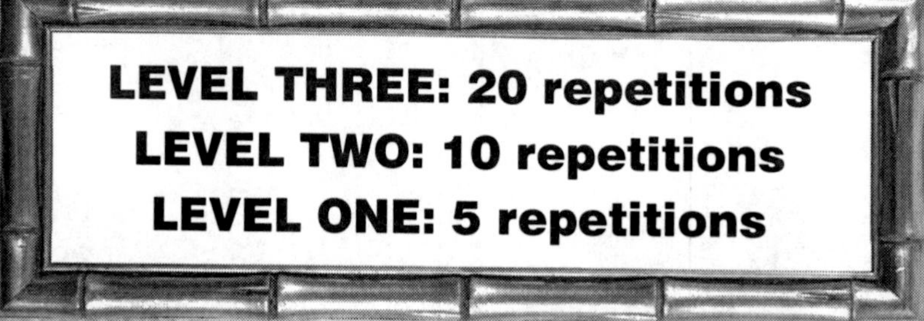
LEVEL THREE: 20 repetitions
LEVEL TWO: 10 repetitions
LEVEL ONE: 5 repetitions

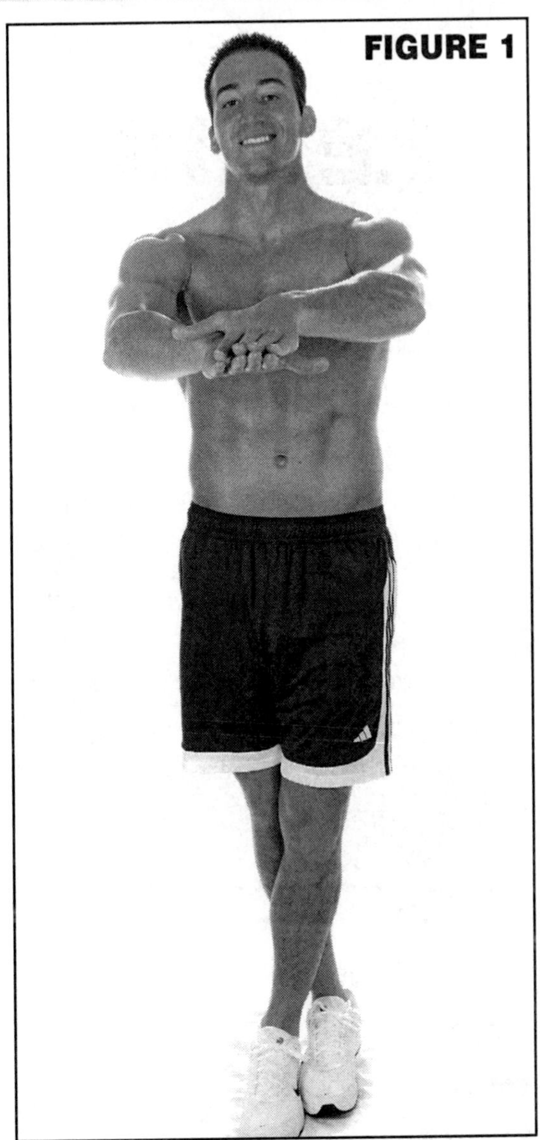
FIGURE 1

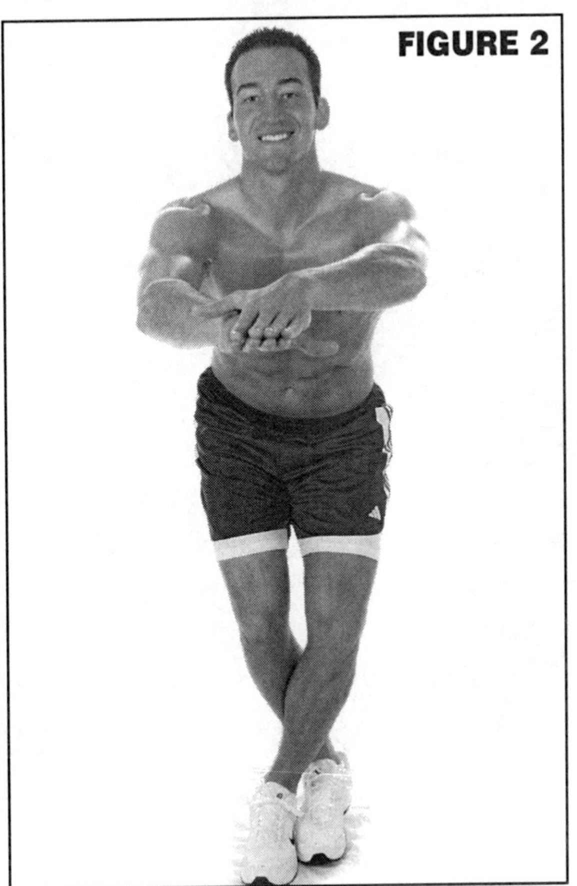
FIGURE 2

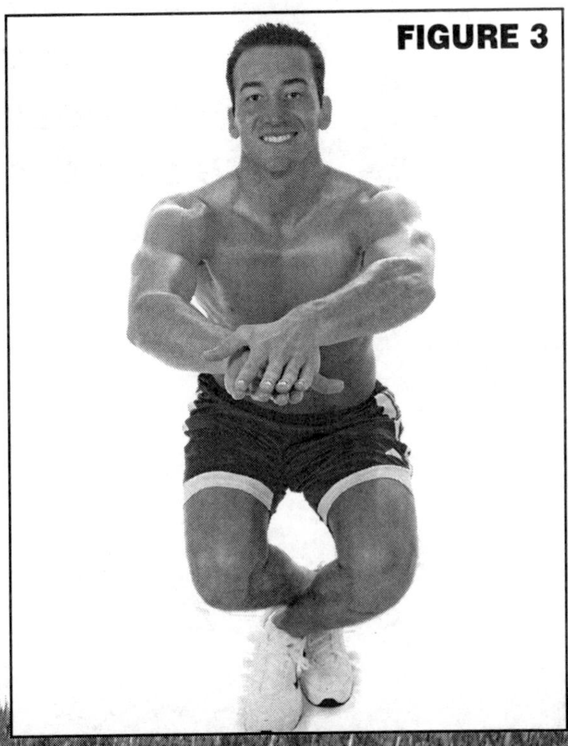
FIGURE 3

#4—FROG FLEX III

Thanks to its webbed feet and powerful legs, the frog is an excellent swimmer—so excellent that militaries around the world refer to their scuba divers as "frogmen." Your next PowerFlex® simulates the up-and-down movement of the frog's legs as it kicks through the water. We'll work the right leg first.

Stand with your feet shoulder-width apart. You may place your hand on your hips or move your arms as if your taking a physical step as illustrated to get added torque on your back leg. Without moving your left foot, step back with your right foot. Keep your right leg straight and rest the ball of your right foot on the floor. Bend your left knee slightly. Keeping your right leg straight, push down on the floor with your right foot and lean forward on to your bent left leg. Hold this position for a second or two. Straighten your left leg and repeat. Reverse the movement to work your left leg. Concentrate on your back leg as this is the one you want to be working, as you want to push the ball of your foot into the floor as hard as you can.

LEVEL THREE: 40 reps (20 per leg)
LEVEL TWO: 20 repetitions
LEVEL ONE: 10 repetitions

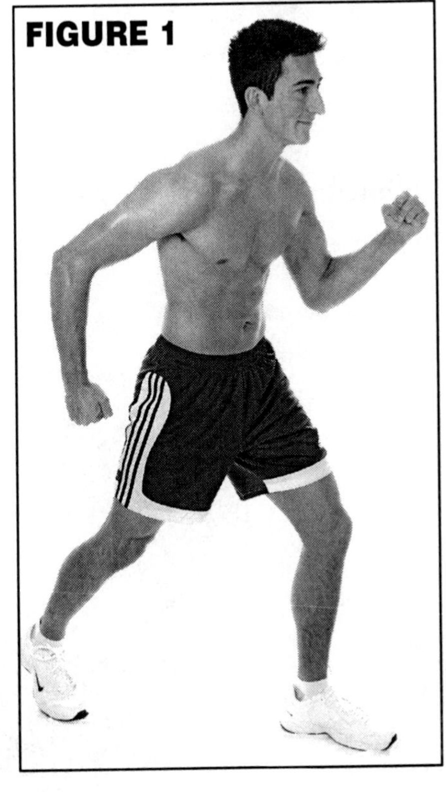
FIGURE 1

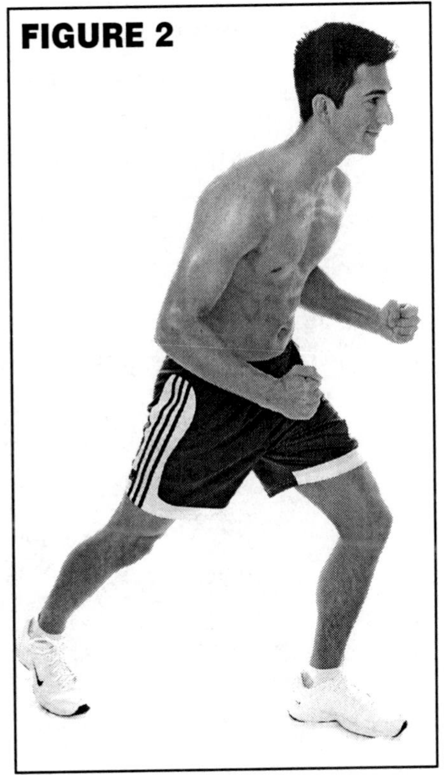
FIGURE 2

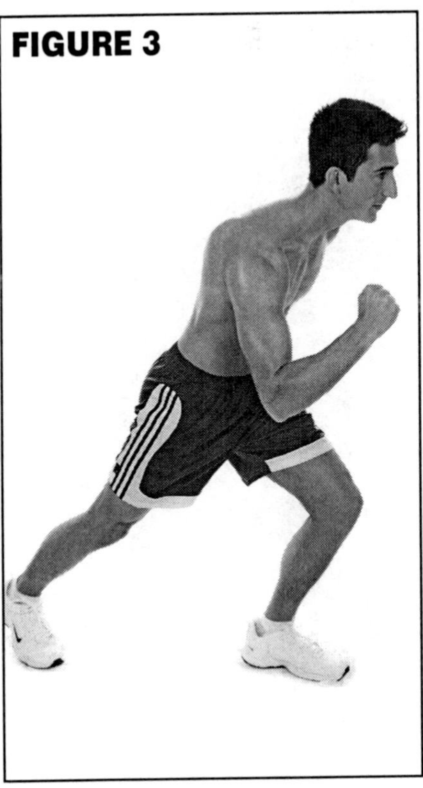
FIGURE 3

#5—KANGAROO FLEX II

Not only does the kangaroo kick with ferocious power, but also with remarkable flexibility and control. This three-part kicking PowerFlex® will help you develop these qualities.

Part One: stand with your feet shoulder-width apart. Your arms hang at your sides, or you can hang on to a chair for balance. Step backward with your right leg, then kick your right leg forward and as high as you can without straining. Keep you right leg straight as you kick. Repeat the movement, kicking with your left leg.

Part Two: same starting position as in Part One. This time, kick your right leg upward and to the left, swinging it from left to right in a circular motion.

Part Three: same starting position as in Parts One and Two. Now, kick your right leg upward and to the right, swinging it from right to left in a circular motion.

Friend, there you have it—a complete Wild Workout® to strengthen, shape, and add power every muscle in your legs, from your toes to your thighs. With consistency and determination you will develop legs that will carry you with confidence, whether you're wearing a football uniform, a business suit, or a bathing suit. See yourself achieving your goals, and see how Wild Workout® helps you achieve them!

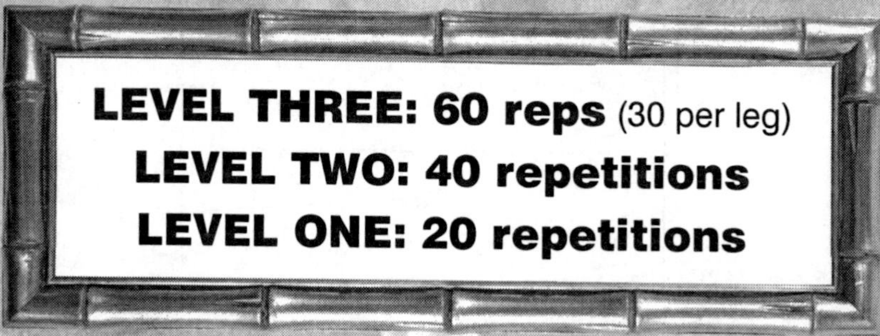

LEVEL THREE: 60 reps (30 per leg)
LEVEL TWO: 40 repetitions
LEVEL ONE: 20 repetitions

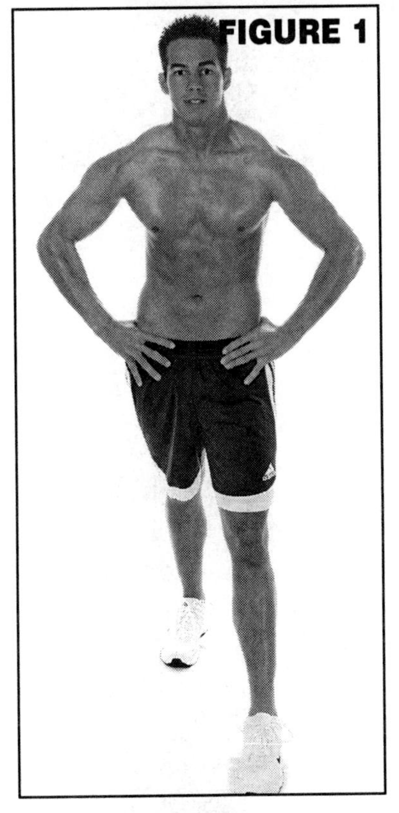
FIGURE 1

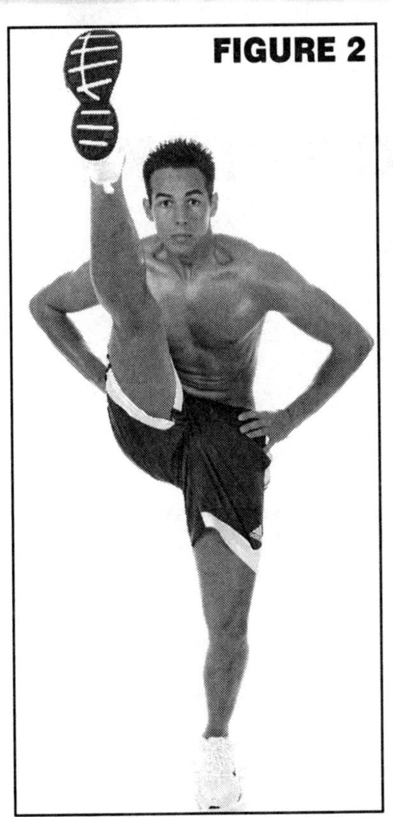
FIGURE 2

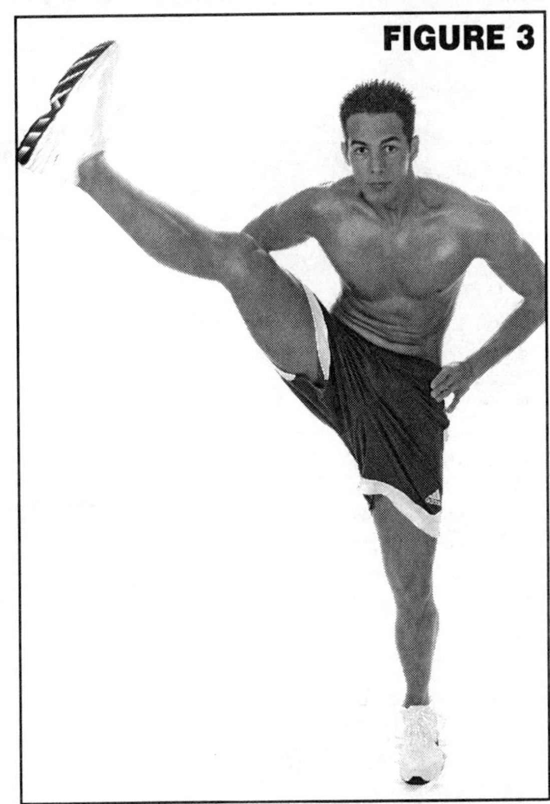
FIGURE 3

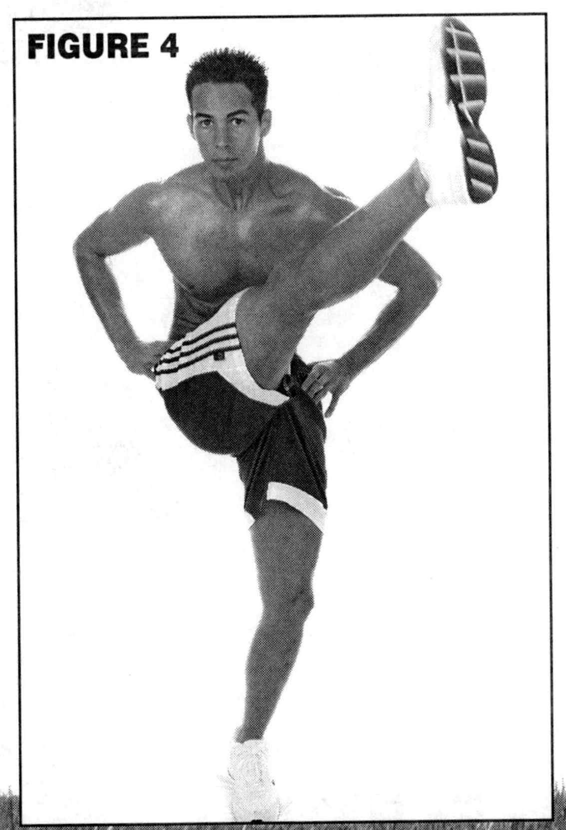
FIGURE 4

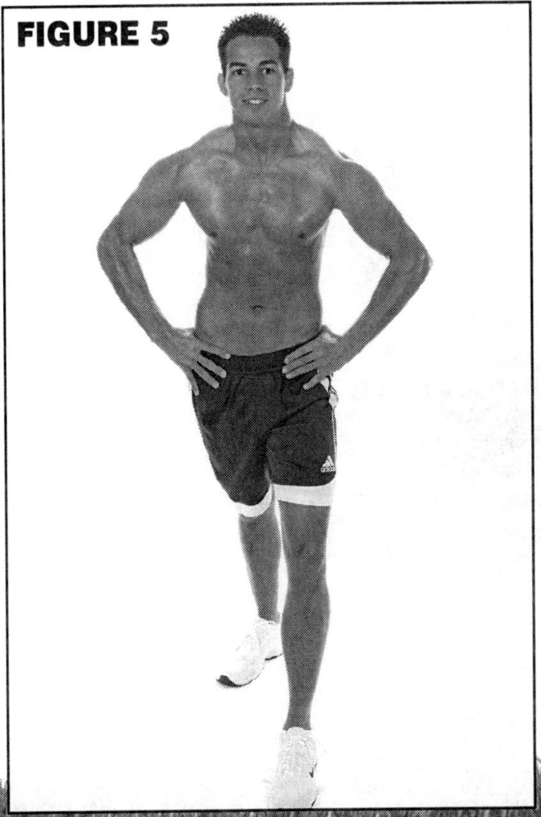
FIGURE 5

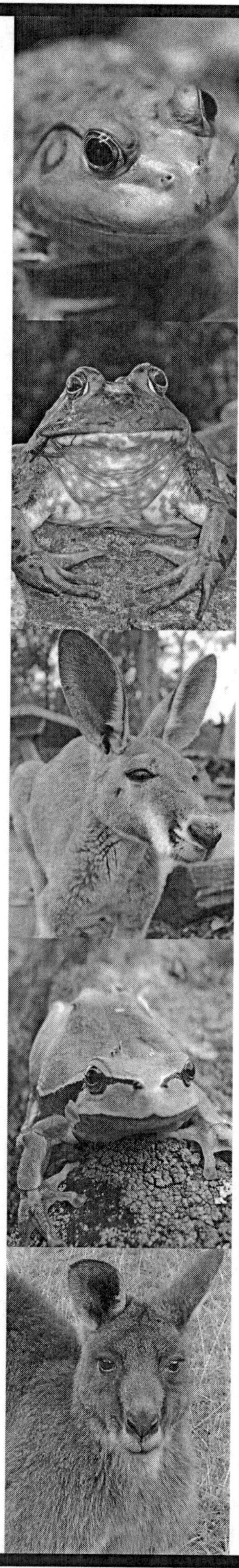

Leg Exercises

FROG FLEX I

FROG FLEX II

KANGAROO FLEX I

FROG FLEX III

KANGAROO FLEX II

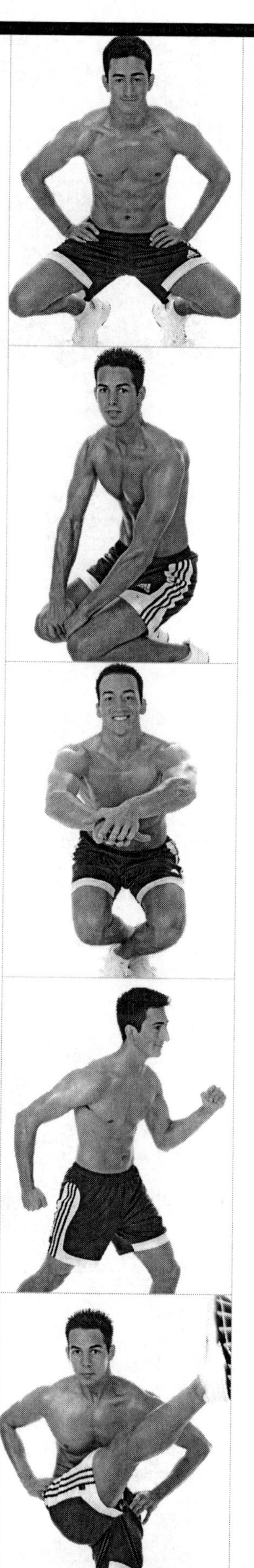

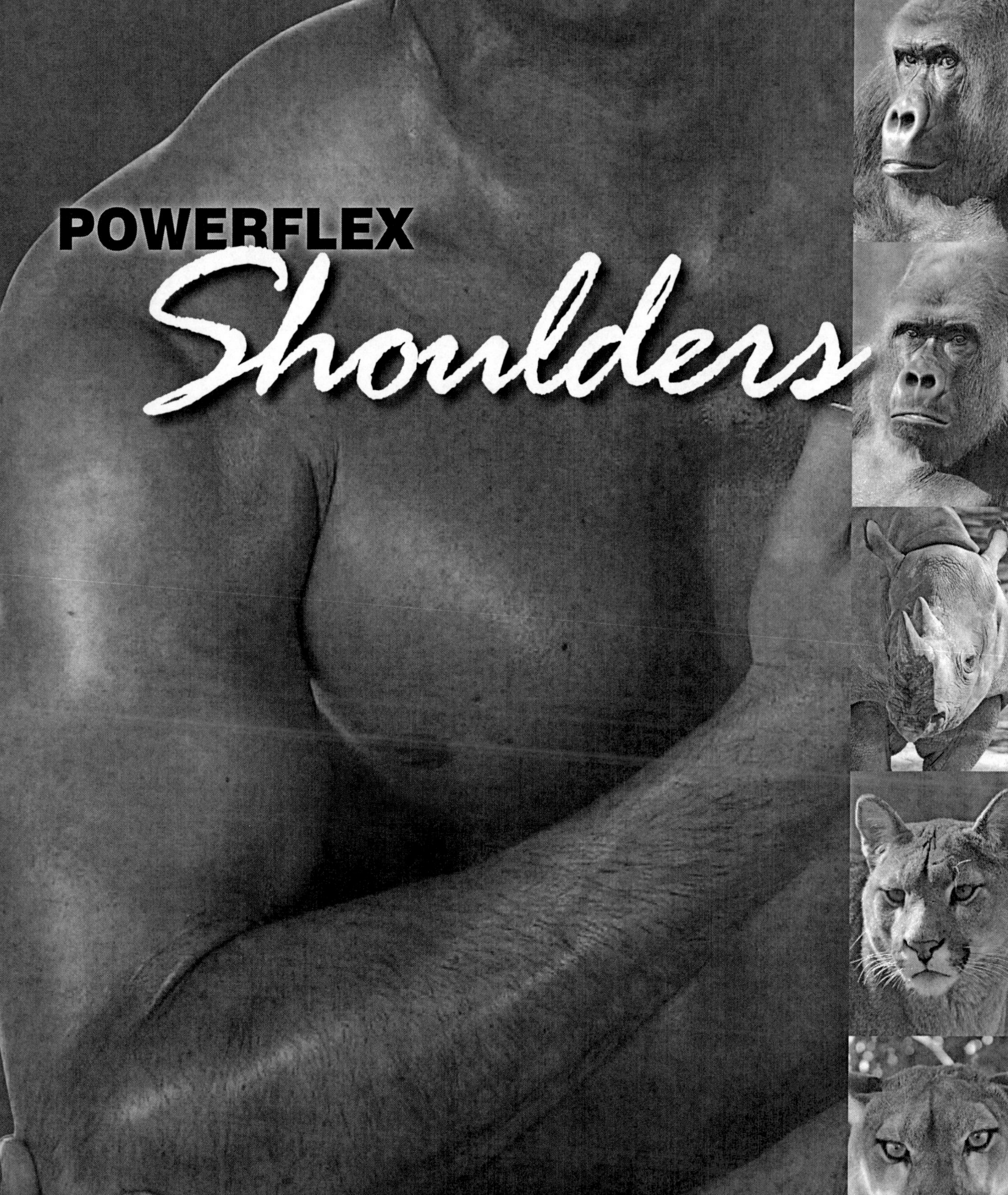
POWERFLEX
Shoulders

SHOULDERS WORKOUT

You can have well-rounded, powerful, healthy shoulders without using equipment, weights, pulleys, or machines. Just do five PowerFlexes for 20 minutes a day.

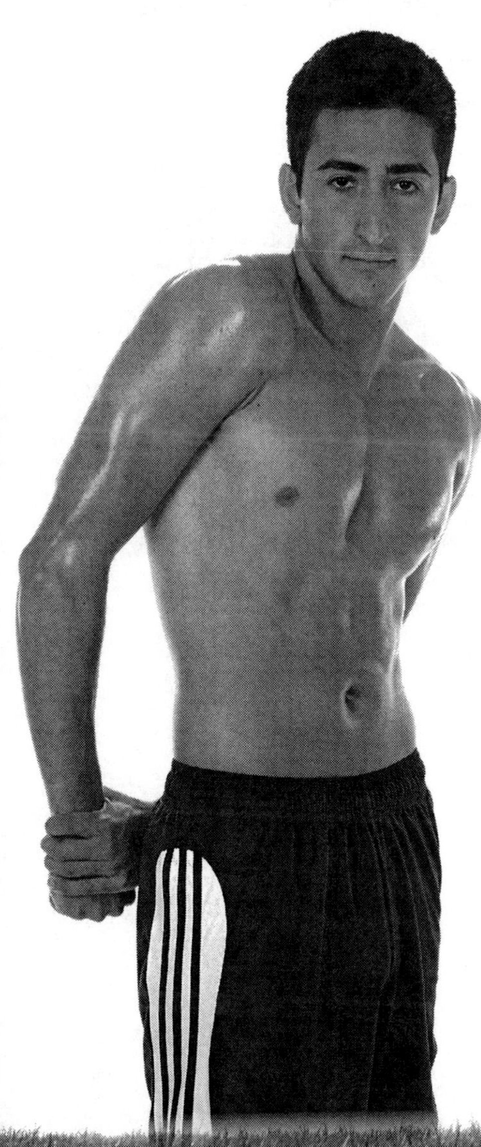

Wild Workout® for Well-Rounded, Powerful,Healthy Shoulders

Shoulders play a vital part in a good looking build. A well defined muscular shapely physique topped off with a pair of well rounded muscular shoulders brings it all together. Developing good healthy shoulders will give you a definite advantage and attraction that is many times overlooked or just skipped over.

It's no coincidence that sayings like "It feels like I'm carrying the weight of the world on my shoulders" puts an emphasis on the shoulders. The shoulders are very crucial when it comes to being able to stand up to the pressure, bear the load, and come out in victory instead of being crumbled in defeat! Not only are shoulder crucial for raw strength and power, in the sense of lowering a shoulder and knocking a door off its hinges, but well toned developed shoulders also offer a side of tenderness and compassion that makes a real bond with others. Lending a shoulder to cry on so to speak. The gorilla has tremendous shoulders, well developed, powerful and well rounded. The fear that grips a person as they witness the awesome strength and power of the gorilla quickly turns to tenderness as they see that same creature bear the weight of their young on their shoulders with care and compassion as they go about their activities. Well rounded, powerful, healthy shoulders are a major attraction also on the magnificent rhino and big cats as well. Now let's get WILD!

#1—GORILLA FLEX II

This PowerFlex® is similar to a gorilla using its fist to push something away. Sit or stand. Bend your right arm at the elbow until your forearm is parallel to the floor. Make a fist with your right hand and place your left palm over your fist. Slowly and smoothly push your right fist forward while resisting with the left hand. Return to the starting position and repeat. Reverse the movement to work your left shoulder. As with all PowerFlexes pay attention to proper form as you're performing each exercise.

LEVEL THREE: 80 reps (40 per side)
LEVEL TWO: 40 repetitions
LEVEL ONE: 20 repetitions

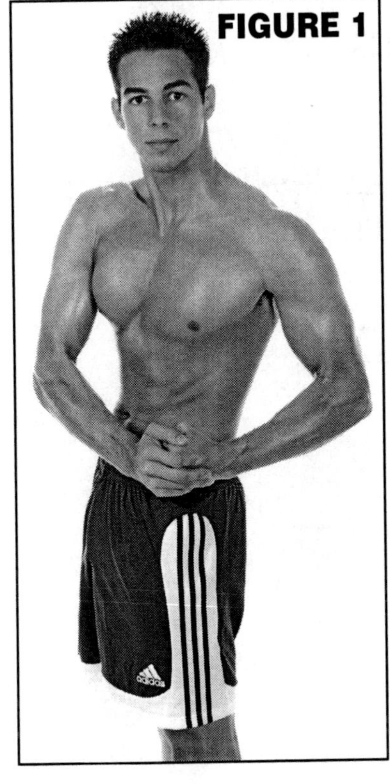
FIGURE 1

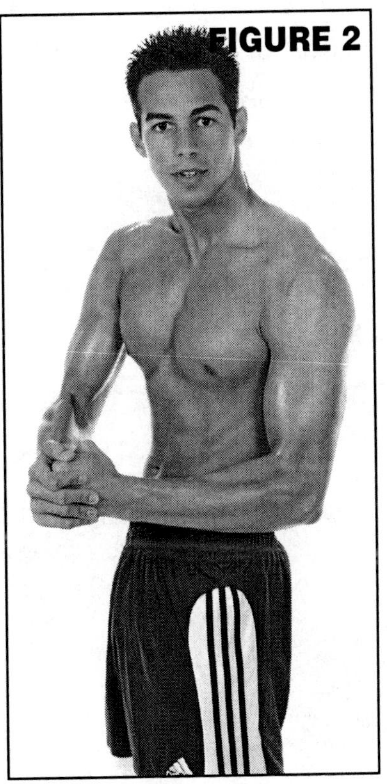
FIGURE 2

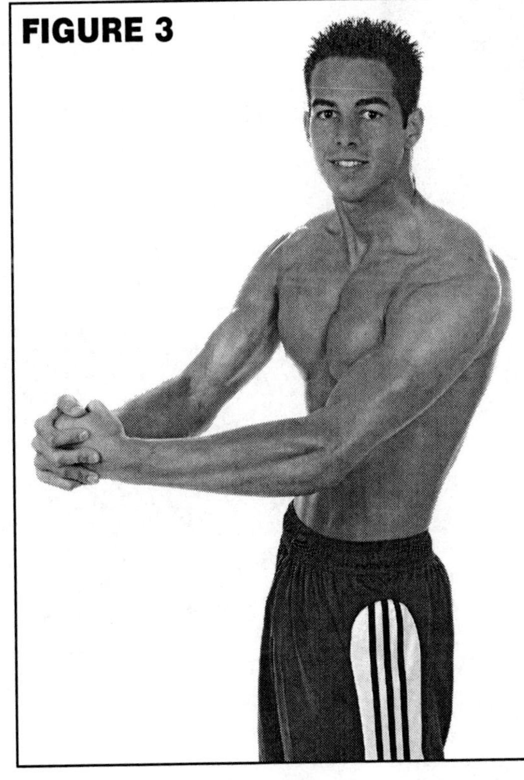
FIGURE 3

#2—GORILLA FLEX III

This PowerFlex® simulates the way the gorilla pulls itself across and up a tree branch as it climbs. Sit or stand. Raise your left elbow until you're holding it across your chest. Place the palm of your right hand under your left elbow. Slowly and smoothly pull your elbow back down to your left side as you resist with your right hand. Return to the starting position and repeat. Reverse the movement to work your right shoulder. The muscles of the front, middle, and rear shoulder allow you to move your arms up, down, and around. Developing strong, impressive shoulders means developing all of these muscles. This PowerFlex® works the rear shoulder muscles.

LEVEL THREE: 60 reps (30 per side)
LEVEL TWO: 40 repetitions
LEVEL ONE: 20 repetitions

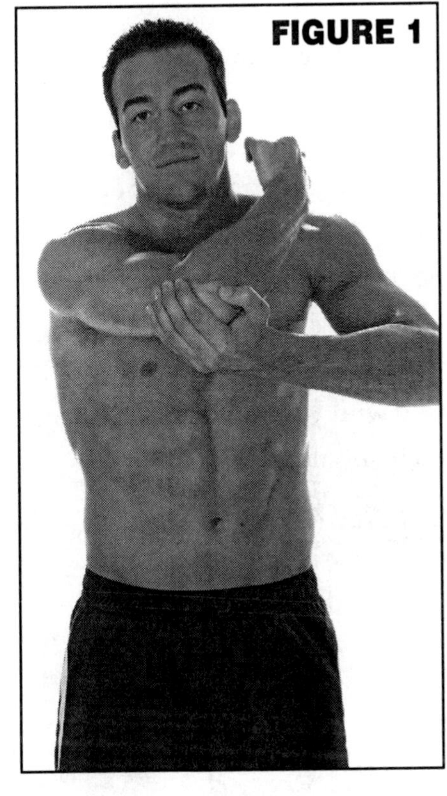
FIGURE 1

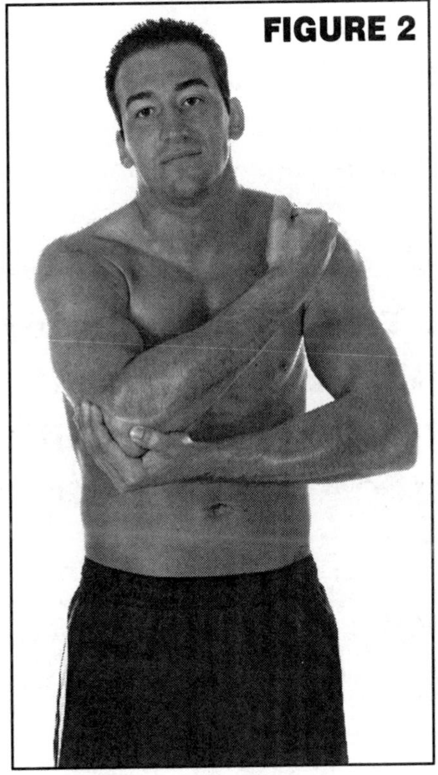
FIGURE 2

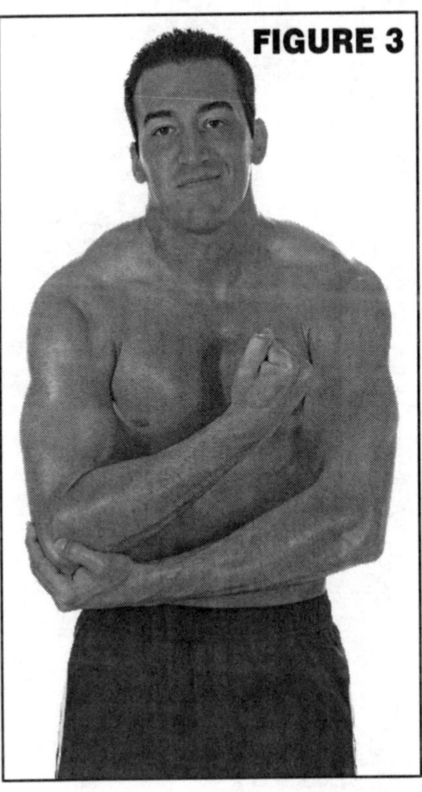
FIGURE 3

#3—RHINO FLEX I

The rhino has strong bulging shoulders, as a matter of fact big game hunters are instructed to shoot for the shoulders, to help bag a trophy. Their shoulders are huge and powerful. Thanks to the immense muscles along the tops of its shoulders, the bulky rhino can pull its legs through deep, sucking mud. Your next PowerFlex® simulates that movement. Concentrate on just working your shoulder, keeping your back straight. Sit or stand. With your left hand, reach behind your back and grasp your right wrist. Slowly and smoothly, raise your right shoulder as high as you can, resisting with your left hand. Return to the starting position and repeat. Reverse the movement to work your left shoulder.

LEVEL THREE: 60 reps (30 per side)
LEVEL TWO: 40 repetitions
LEVEL ONE: 20 repetitions

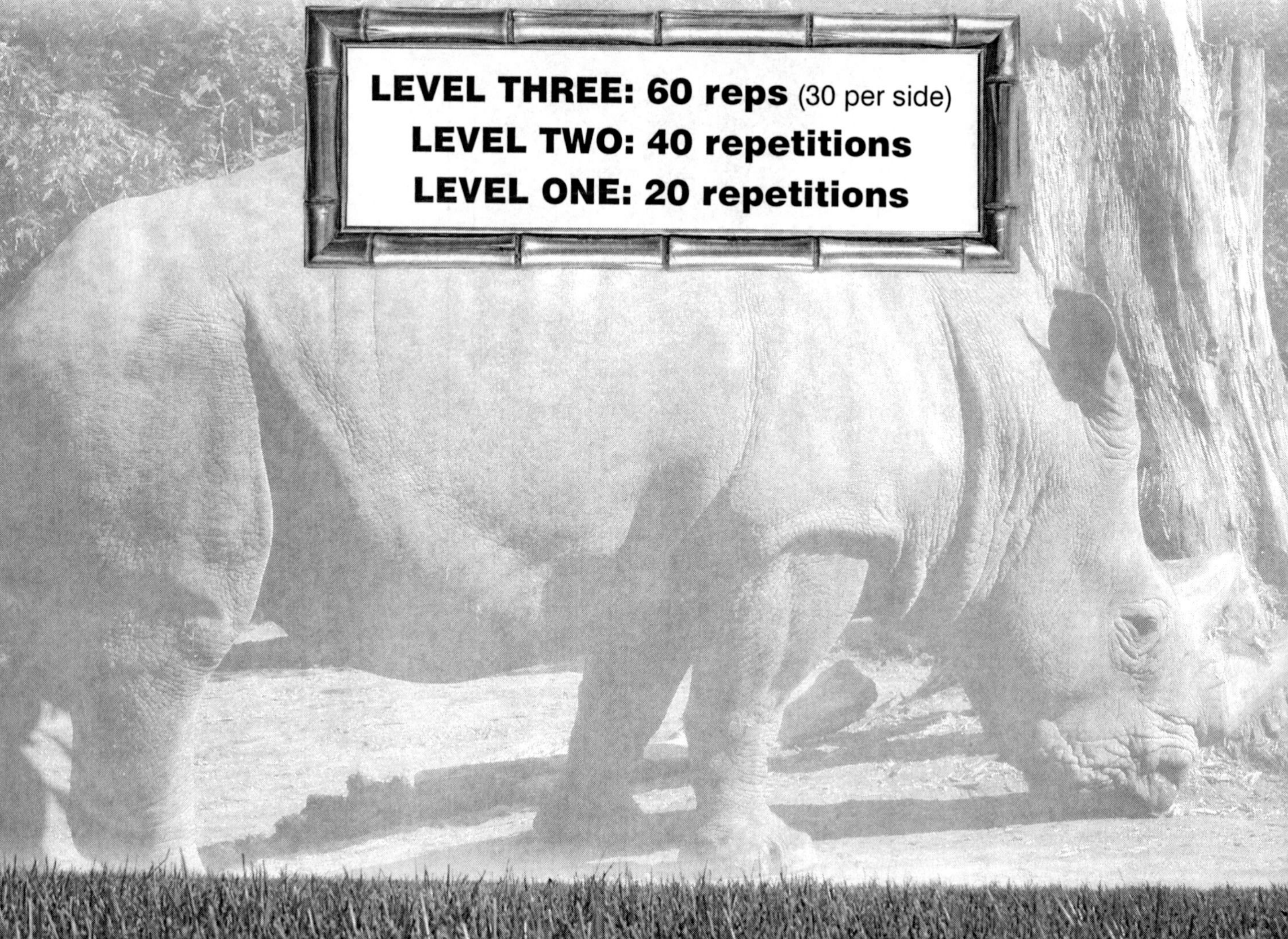

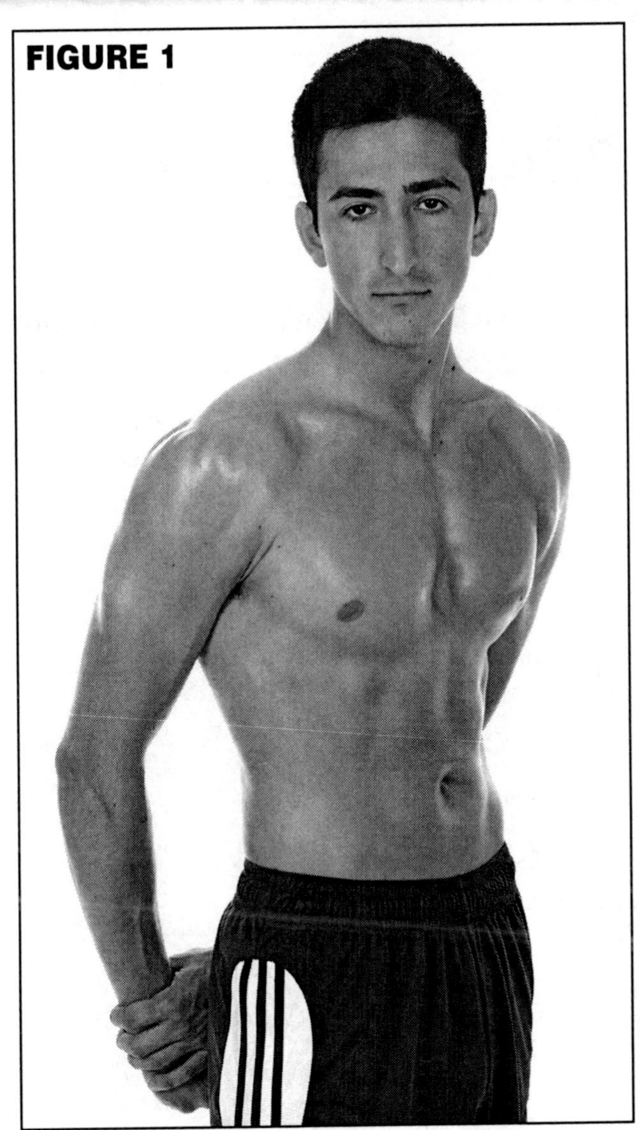

FIGURE 1

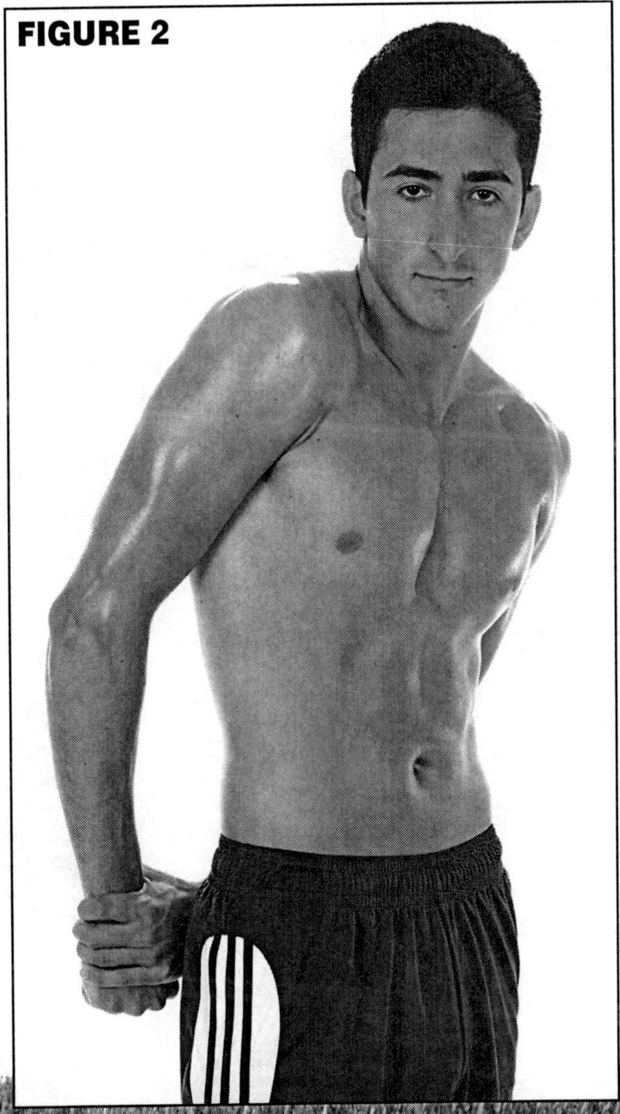

FIGURE 2

#4—COUGAR FLEX I

The cougar is a fearsome predator, moving quietly, then striking with deadly force. Its powerful shoulders allow it to overpower its prey and to wield its sharp claws with pinpoint control. This PowerFlex® simulates that striking movement. It's excellent for developing the middle shoulder muscles. Sit or stand. Raise your right arm across your body just beneath chest level. Your right palm should be facing down. With your left hand, grasp your right wrist. Slowly and smoothly push your right arm up and out while resisting with your left hand. Return to the starting position and repeat. Reverse the movement to work your left shoulder.

LEVEL THREE: 80 reps (40 per side)
LEVEL TWO: 40 repetitions
LEVEL ONE: 20 repetitions

While doing the PowerFlexes you can put a lot of effort and resistance into each movement, or not so much effort and resistance in each movement; according to how you want to develop, and according to what look you want to get. It's truly amazing!

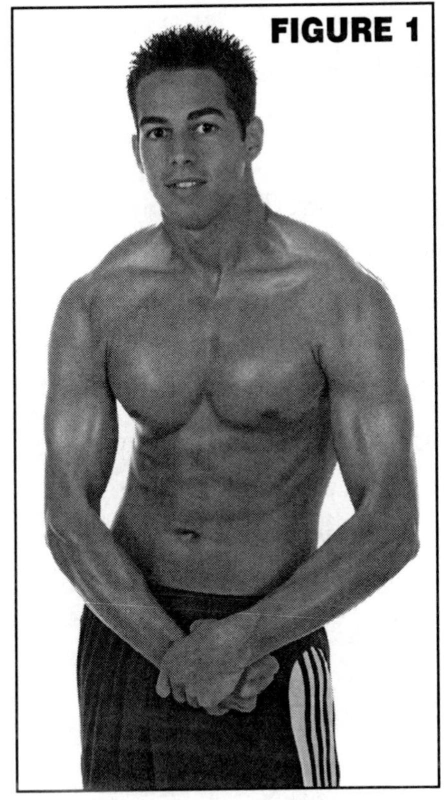
FIGURE 1

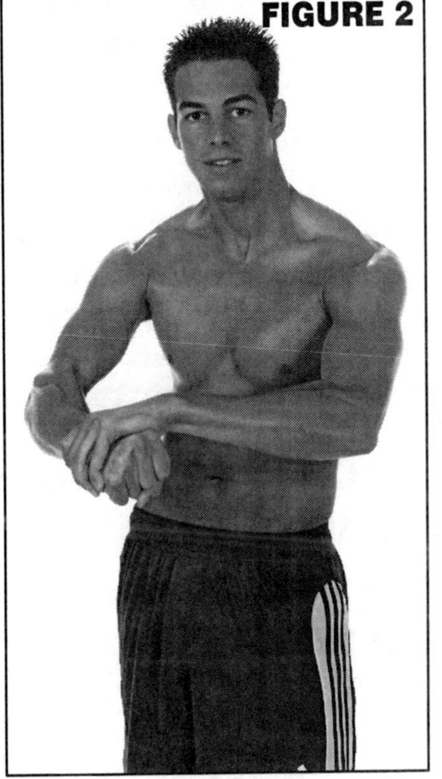
FIGURE 2

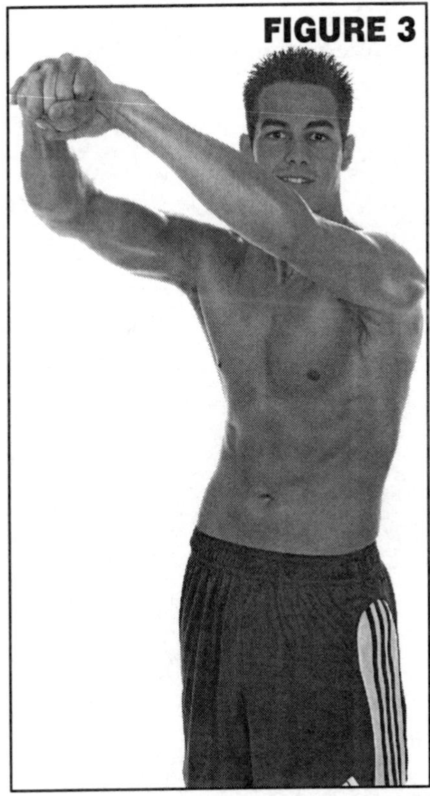
FIGURE 3

#5—COUGAR FLEX II

After taking its prey, the cougar tears its flesh and begins to feed. The last PowerFlex® of this workout simulates that tearing movement—raw power at its max. Sit or stand. Raise your left arm across your stomach. Your left palm should be facing up. With your right hand, grasp your left wrist. Slowly and smoothly pull your left hand back toward your left side while resisting with your right hand. Return to the starting position and repeat. Reverse the movement to work your right shoulder.

That my friend is the Wild Workout® for well rounded, powerful, healthy, muscular shoulders! The next time you hear the phrase "It feels like I'm carrying the weight of the world on my shoulders" you can smile inside knowing that you know just how important the shoulders are. And you have developed yours to carry the load, the next time the world falls down on yours! No get busy! You have found a winner when you found the Wild Workout®, it really works! Now get at it!

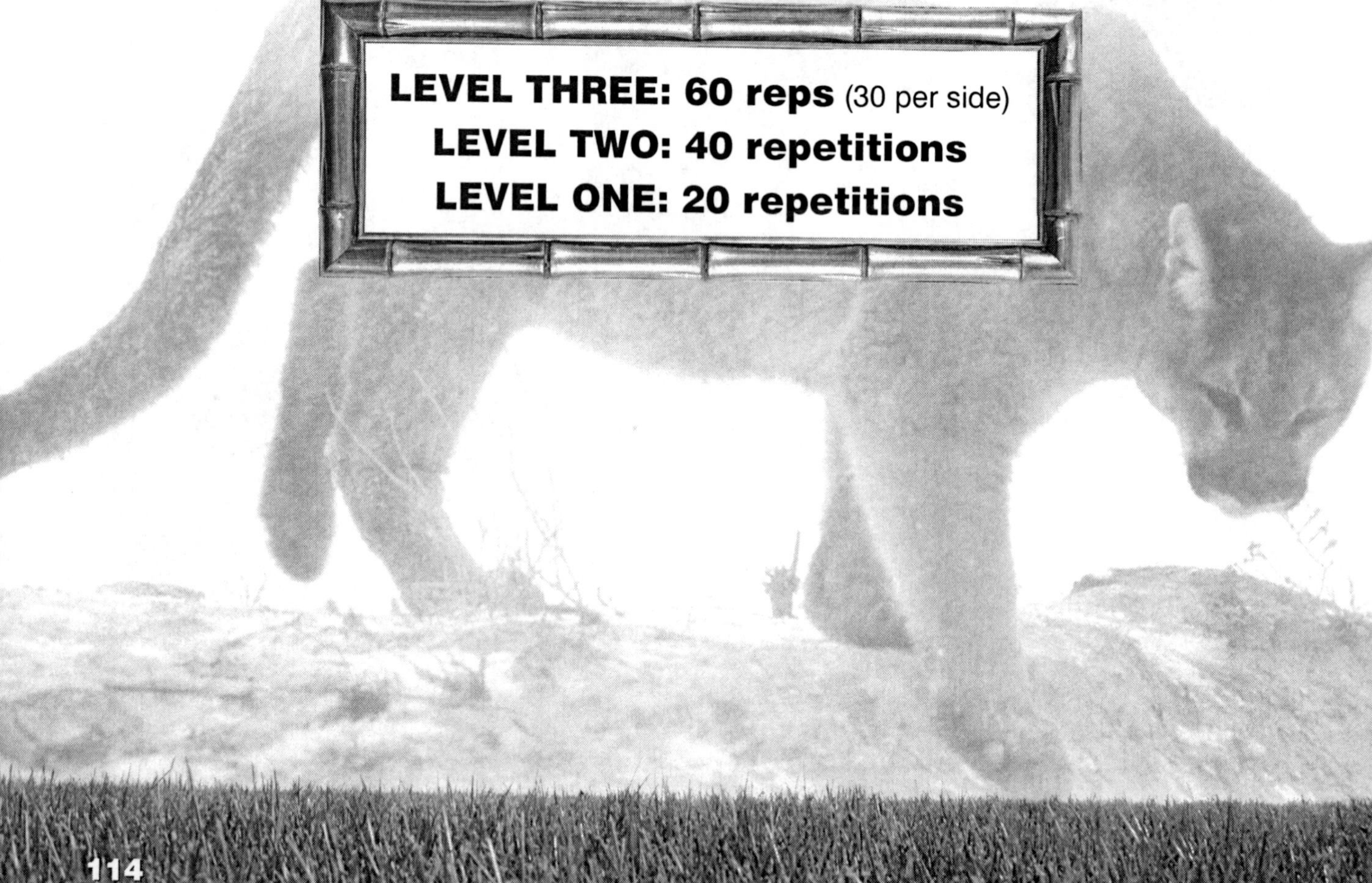

LEVEL THREE: 60 reps (30 per side)
LEVEL TWO: 40 repetitions
LEVEL ONE: 20 repetitions

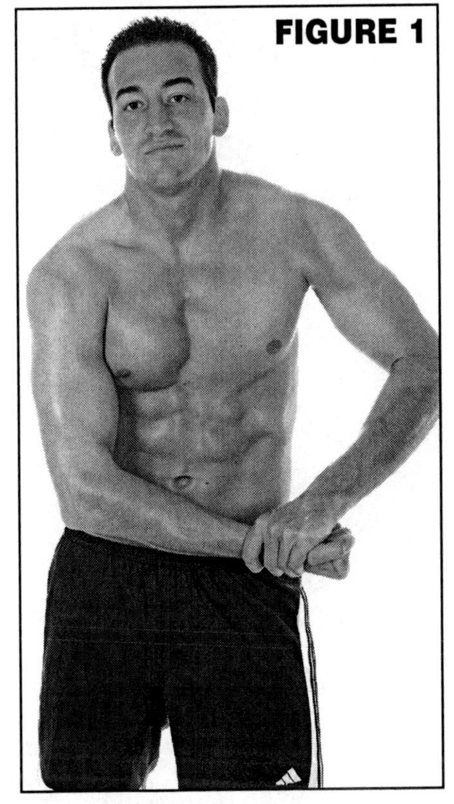
FIGURE 1

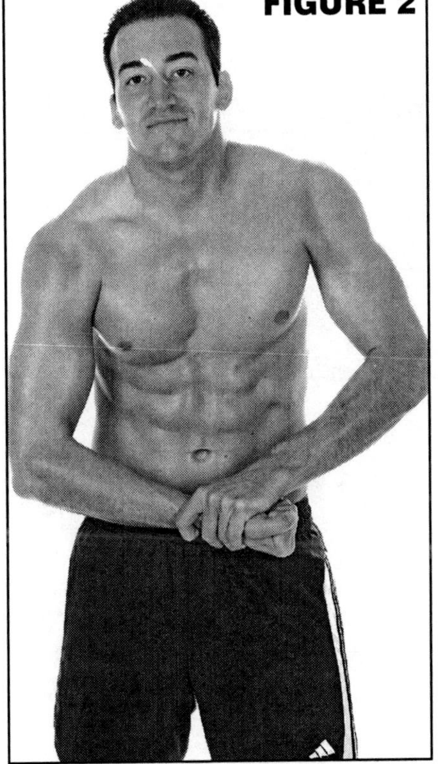
FIGURE 2

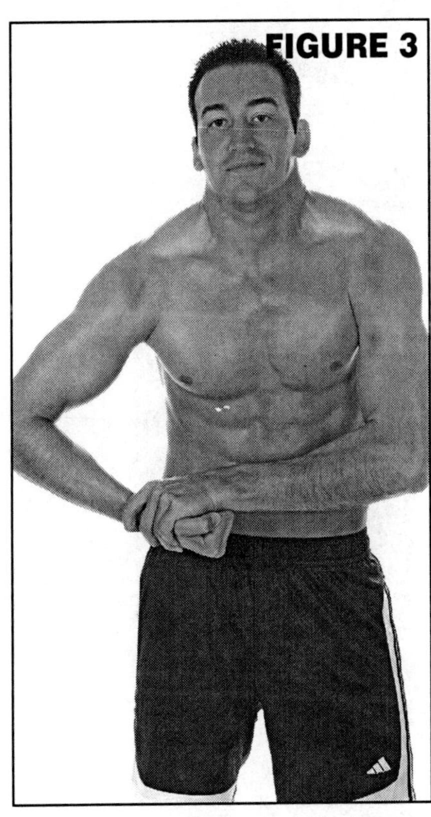
FIGURE 3

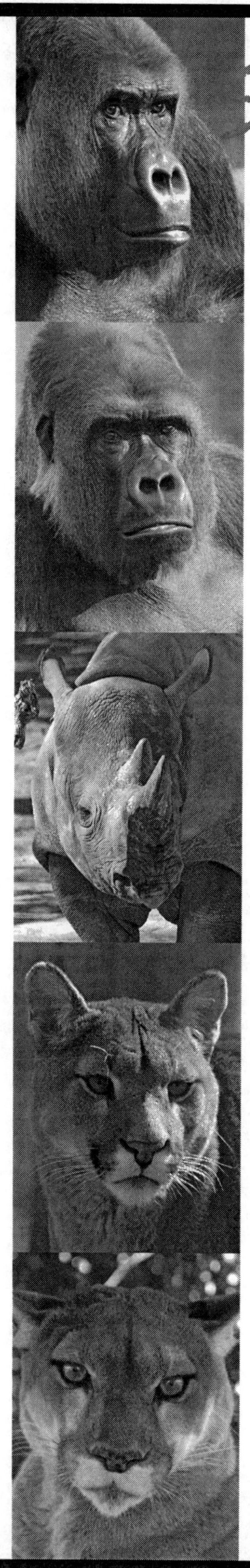

Shoulder Exercises

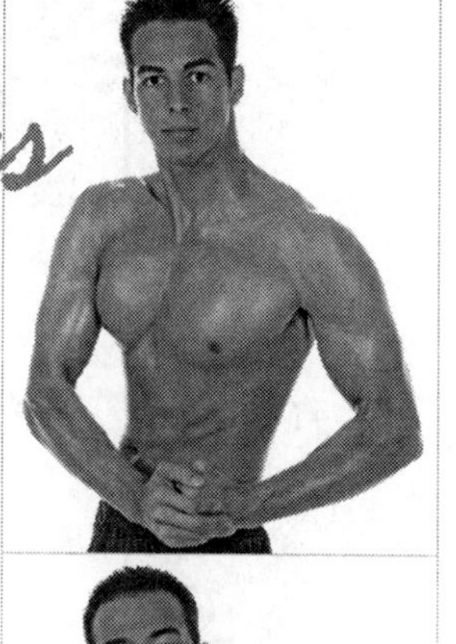

GORILLA FLEX II

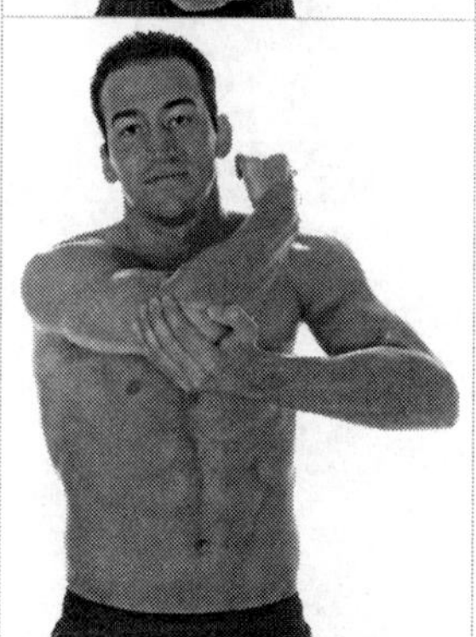

GORILLA FLEX III

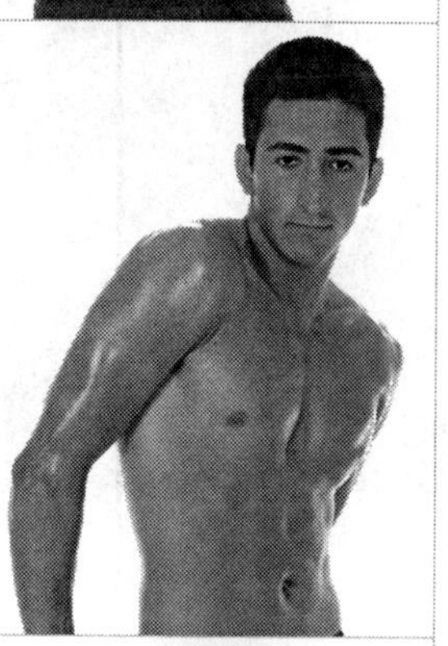

RHINO FLEX I

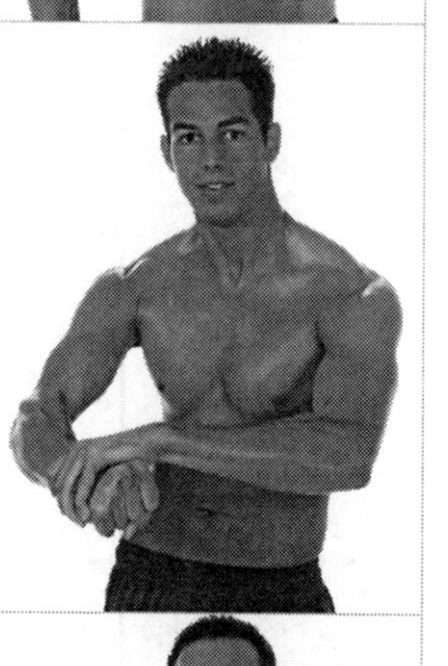

COUGAR FLEX I

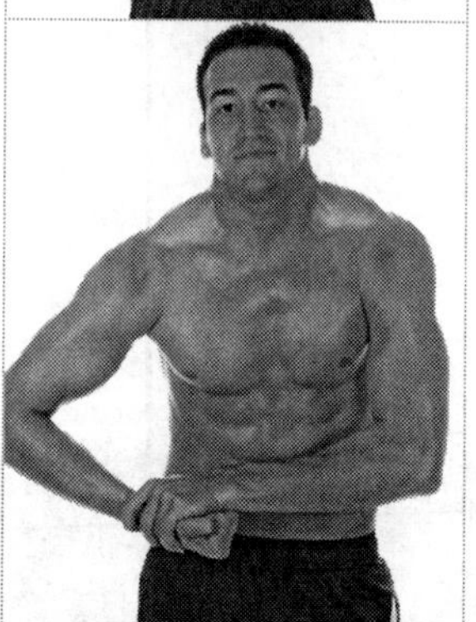

COUGAR FLEX II

POWERFLEX *Arms*

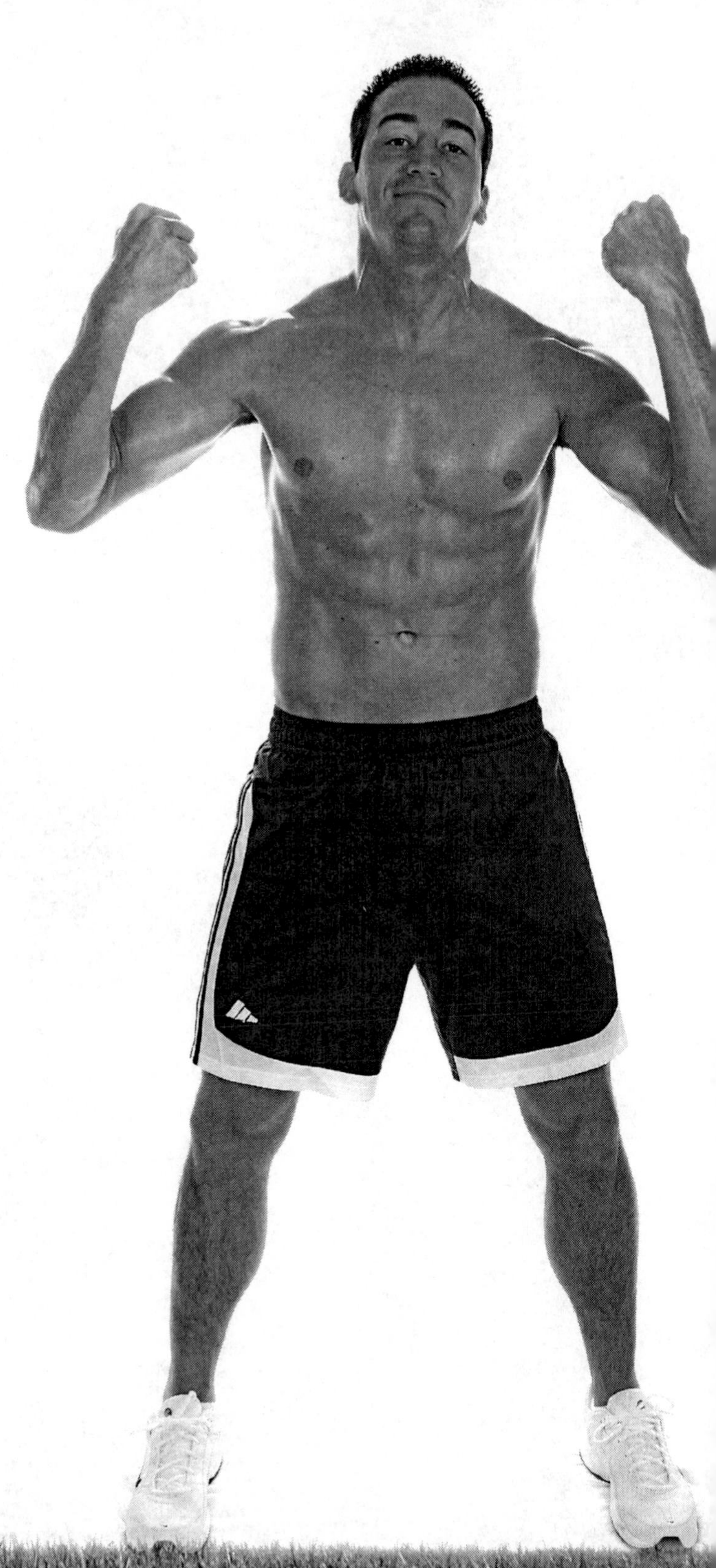

ARMS WORKOUT

You can have strong, muscular, well-shaped, awesome arms without using equipment, weights, pulleys, or machines. Just do five PowerFlexes for 20 minutes a day.

Wild Workout® for Strong, Muscular, Well-Defined Arms

Having well developed arms, filled with muscle and power, is quite an attractive and eye catching sight! The flex of a bulging bicep has always been a way of showing off for the one you want to attract as well as scaring off the others that would move into your territory. Bulging biceps combined with tremendous triceps (muscles in the upper back part of the arm) added to well shaped forearms has always been a symbol of strength, conditioning, and power. Not only are well developed arms an attractive feature to onlookers, but they are also confidence builders to the one who possesses them. When you develop your arms, your self-esteem is also developed, as well as your self confidence, and your overall person image you have of yourself. Having well shaped powerful arms are a real boost!

The good news is the arms are also the muscles that respond the fastest and can be developed so quickly. Some see the fun in quick response of the biceps and triceps and when they develop bulging arm muscles they forget about the rest of the body. Remember the arms are extensions, extremities, branches so to speak of the trunk of the body. The trunk holds all the vital organs; respiratory system, electrical impulses, and also controls the blood flow, and it is so important to work this out. When you see a well developed chest, with rippling abs, a healthy spine, firm neck, strong back, carried about upon shapely powerful legs, highlighted by round muscular shoulders, is when strong well define sculpted arms become the icing on the cake.

When it comes to strong, muscular arms the gorilla reigns as king. It is one of the only animals whose arms are actually stronger than its legs. It is no accident that the movie producers entitled the movie of a giant gorilla King Kong, and struck terror in the audience as its huge arms pounded upon its chest. The arm strength that the gorilla possesses from lifting its entire body weight with one arm as it climbs, to striking its enemies with deadly force it is just too much to begin to list. Many people are complimented when they have big muscular arms by the phrase "Wow, they have arms like a Shaved Ape!"

The big cat family also have powerful arms, the Lion, Tiger, Jaguar, Cougar, the power in their front legs are awesome! Some recorded that the lion is powerful enough to drag an elephant with one paw. Now let's get onto the Wild Workout® for muscular, sculpted, and powerful arms. Let's get WILD!

#1—GORILLA FLEX IV

The gorilla has inspired five of the PowerFlexes in this course. You did the first one in the Chest Workout, the second and third ones in the Arm workout, and here's number four. To build impressive arms, it's important to work the biceps, triceps, and forearms from many different angles. This unique PowerFlex® works the biceps from two angles.

Part One: sit or stand, with your right arm hanging at your side and your right hand palm up. With your left hand, grasp your right wrist. Slowly and smoothly bend your right elbow and pull your right hand toward your shoulder as you resist with your left hand. Lower your right hand and repeat. Reverse the movement to work your left arm.

Part Two: same starting position as Part One. Reach behind your back with your left hand and grasp your right wrist. Slowly and smoothly, bend your right elbow and pull your right hand toward your shoulder as you resist with your left hand. Lower your right hand and repeat. Reverse the movement to work your left arm.

You may find part two to be a little difficult to do. Try to let the elbow of the working arm move back and pull your hand toward your armpit as far as you can without straining.

LEVEL THREE: 60 reps (15 per arm)
LEVEL TWO: 40 repetitions
LEVEL ONE: 20 repetitions

FIGURE 1

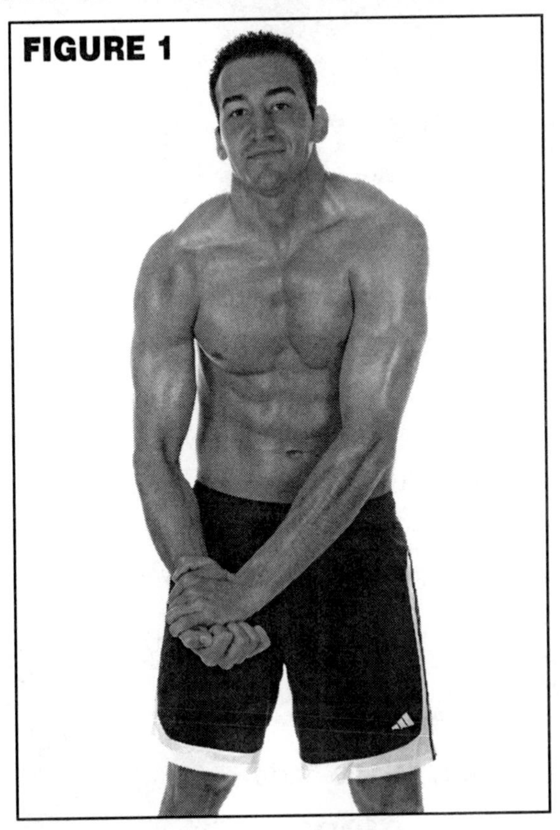

FIGURE 2

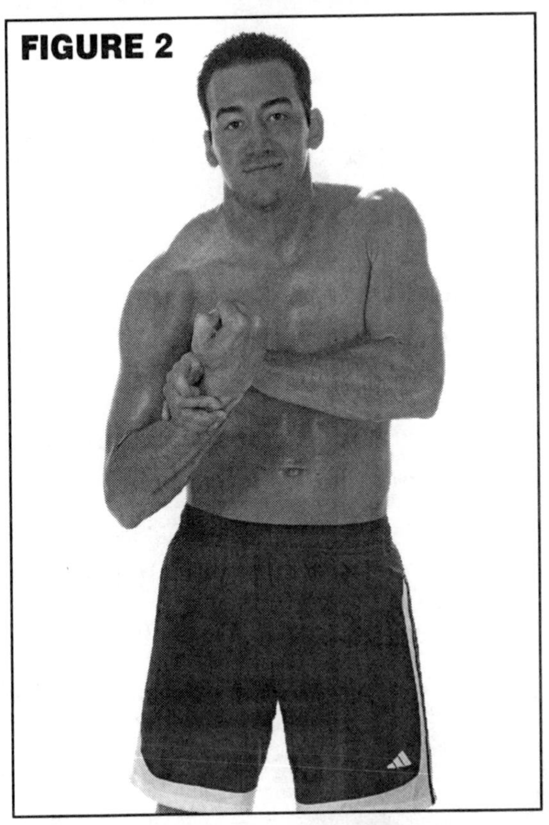

FIGURE 3

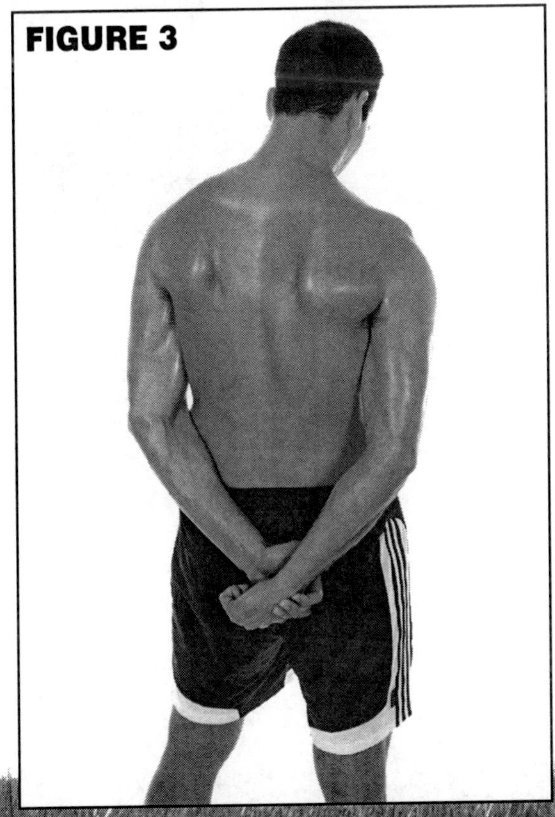

FIGURE 4

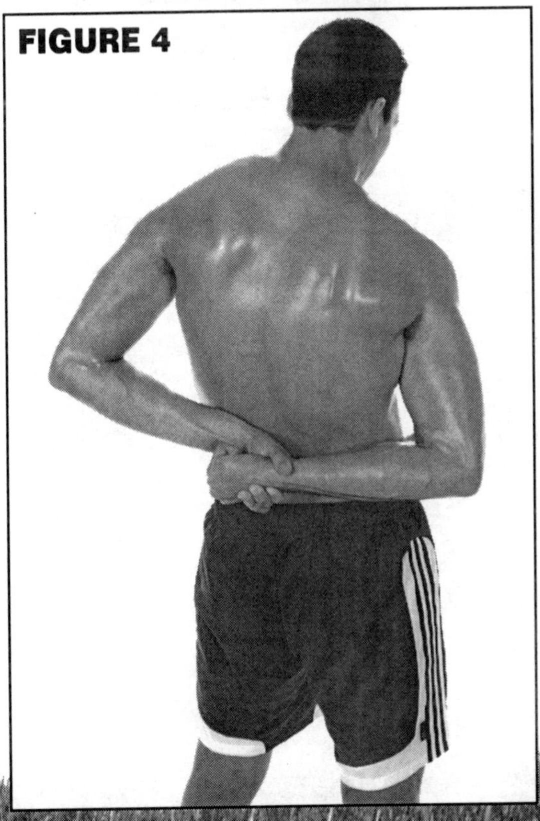

#2—LION FLEX I

The lion's incredible speed and strength allow it to overcome animals much larger than itself, like the elephant and the water buffalo. Your next PowerFlex® (for the triceps) simulates the way the lion reaches out to slash its prey.

Sit or stand, with your right arm hanging at your side. Make a fist with your right hand. Bend your right elbow and pull your right hand toward your shoulder. With your left hand, grasp your right fist from beneath. Keeping your right elbow close to your side, slowly and smoothly push your right hand down and out as you resist with your left hand. Raise your right hand and repeat. Reverse the movement to work your left arm.

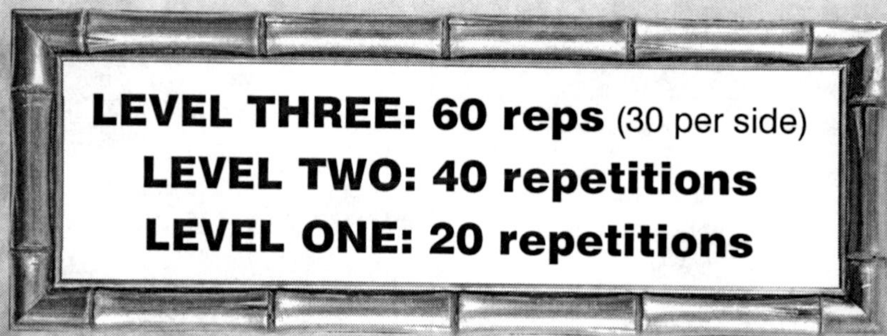

LEVEL THREE: 60 reps (30 per side)
LEVEL TWO: 40 repetitions
LEVEL ONE: 20 repetitions

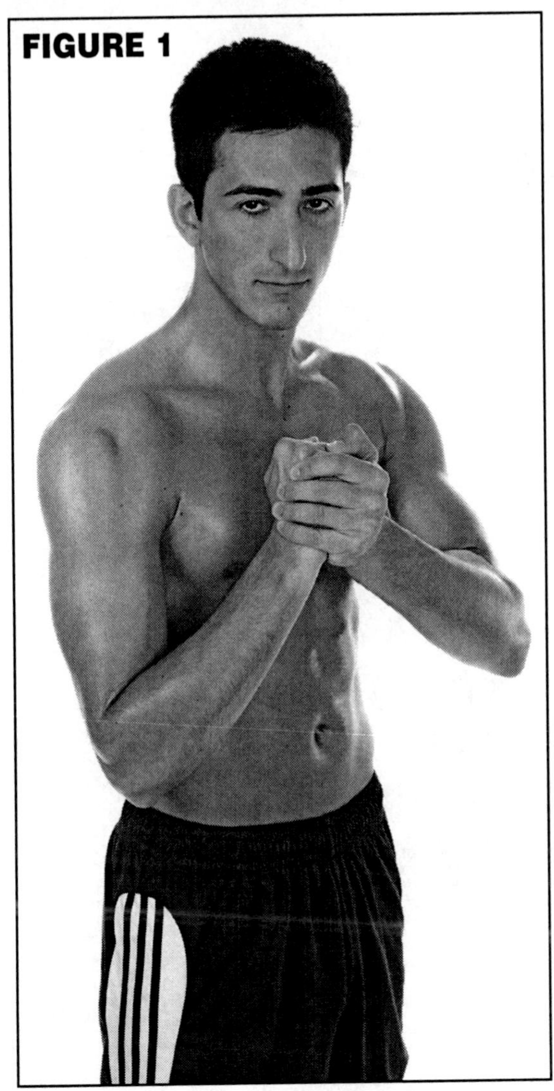
FIGURE 1

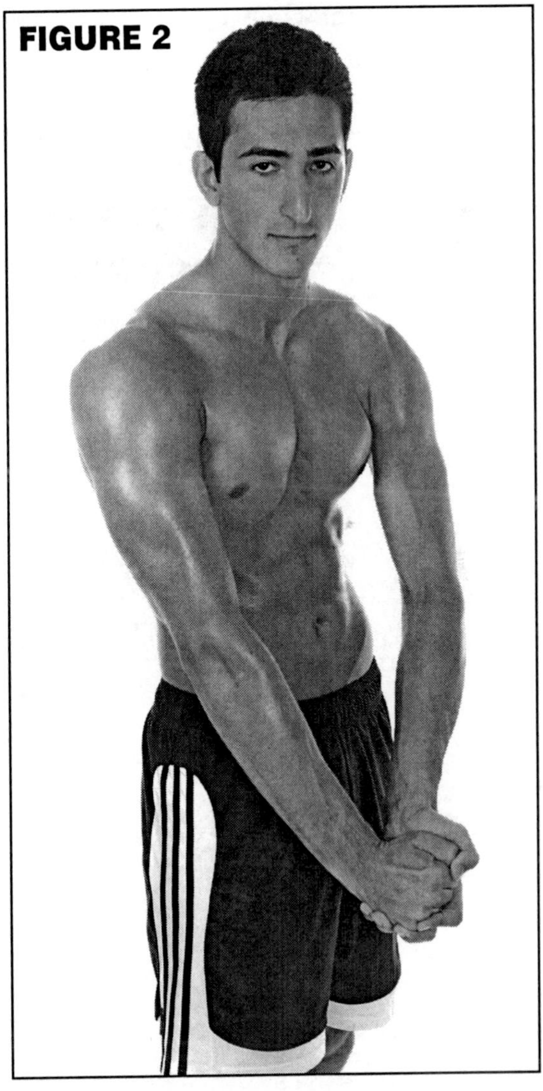
FIGURE 2

#3—TIGER FLEX I

Like the lion, the tiger is feared for its lightning-fast strikes and razor-sharp claws. Similar to Lion Flex I, this next PowerFlex® also works the triceps, but from a different angle.

Sit or stand. Raise your right arm and hold it across your chest. With your left hand, grasp the back of your right wrist. Keeping your right upper arm close to your side, slowly and smoothly push your right forearm up and out while resisting with your left hand. Return to the starting position and repeat. Reverse the movement to work your left arm.

LEVEL THREE: 40 reps (20 per side)
LEVEL TWO: 20 repetitions
LEVEL ONE: 10 repetitions

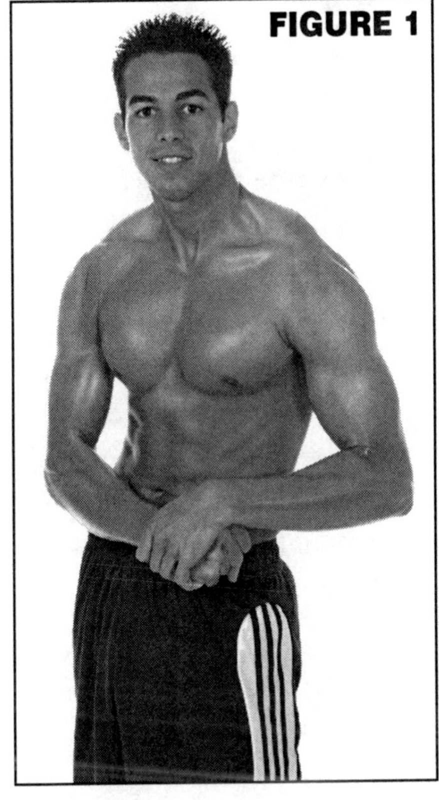
FIGURE 1

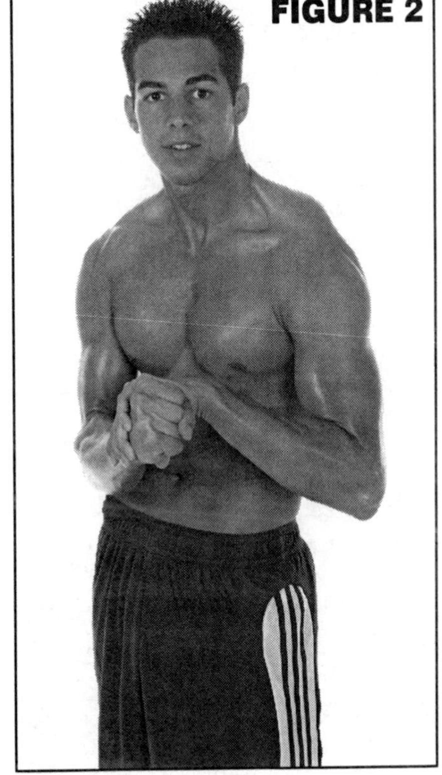
FIGURE 2

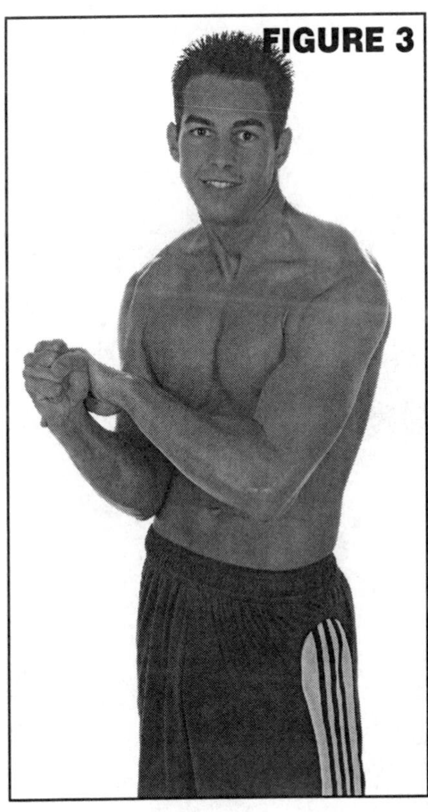
FIGURE 3

#4—JAGUAR FLEX I

It's amazing to watch slow-motion film of a running jaguar. With every stride, the jaguar pulls itself forward, then stretches its legs, grasps the ground with its feet, and pulls again. This Power-Flex® simulates these movements and works the biceps, triceps, and forearms all at once.

Sit or stand, with your arms hanging at your sides. With your thumbs facing forward, make your hands into tight fists. Slowly and smoothly, bend both of your arms at the elbows and twist your fists until your palms are facing the tops of your shoulders (as though you're a bodybuilder doing a "double biceps" pose). Lower your arms slowly and smoothly. When you return to the starting position, push back on your arms (as though you're trying to bend them backward at the elbows) for a second or two. Repeat. Keep your fists tight and feel the tension in your forearms. As you raise your fists, feel the tension in your biceps. As you lower your fists and push back on your arms, feel the tension in your triceps.

LEVEL THREE: 20 repetitions
LEVEL TWO: 10 repetitions
LEVEL ONE: 5 repetitions

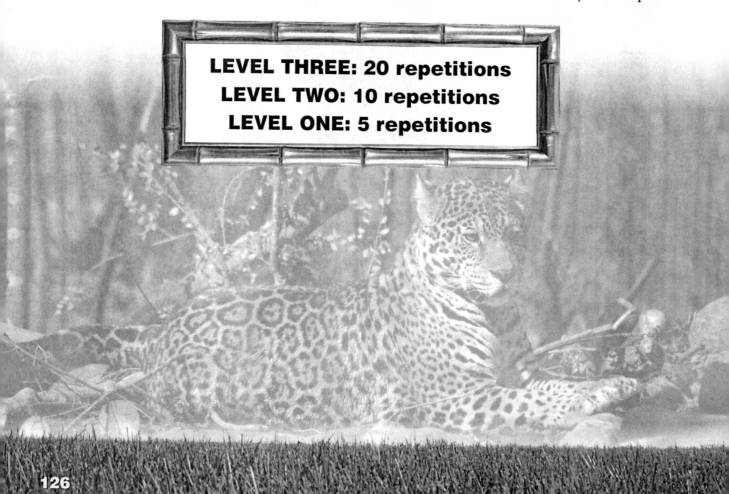

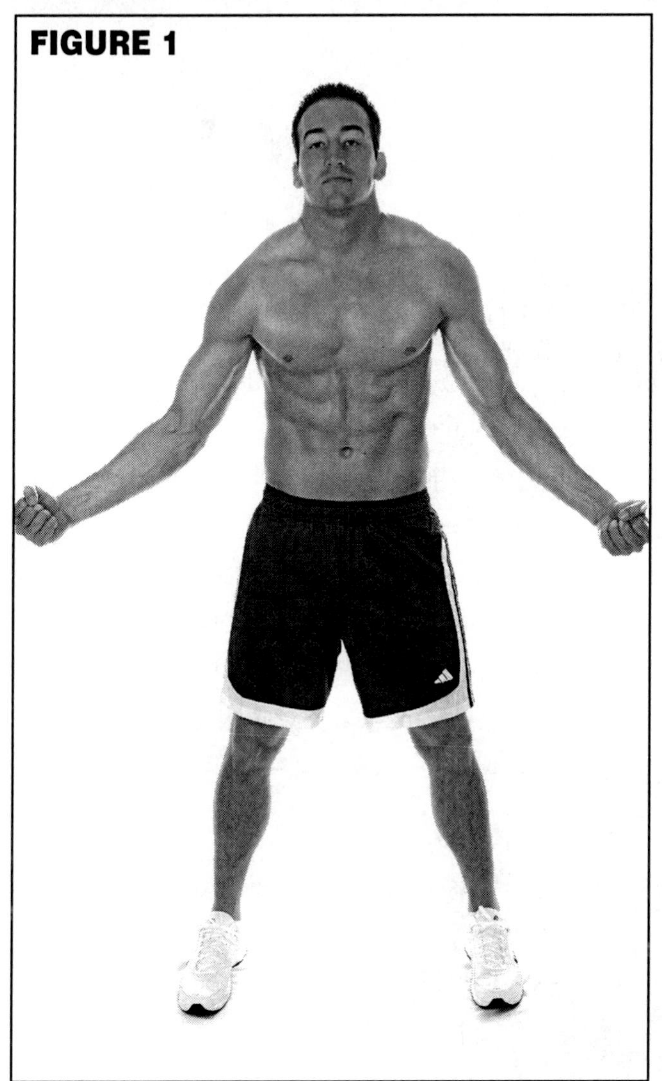

FIGURE 1

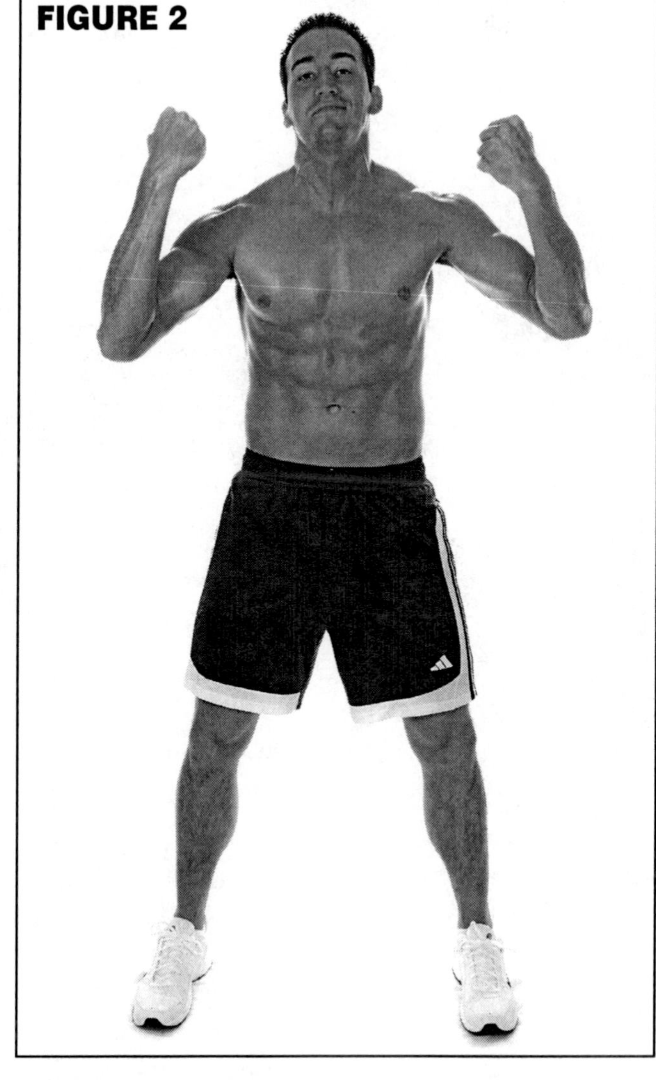

FIGURE 2

#5—GORILLA FLEX V

This Gorilla Flex is a fine all-in-one PowerFlex® for your biceps, triceps, and forearms.

Part One: sit or stand, with your arms hanging at your sides. Your hands should be open with the palms facing your sides, like an aggressive gorilla boldly staking his claim getting ready for action if needs be. Push back on your arms (as you did for Jaguar Flex I) for a second or two. Now shake the tension out of your arms and relax for a few moments.

Part Two: next, make a fist with your right hand. Bend your right arm at the elbow and twist your fist until your palm is facing the top of your right shoulder (as you did with both arms for Jaguar Flex I). Hold this position for a second or two, then relax your right arm.

Part Three: same as for Part Two, but reverse the movement to work your left arm. One cycle through all three parts counts as one repetition.

There you go, friend—a complete Wild Workout® for building arms that mean business. Thanks to the strong foundation you've built through practicing the previous Workouts, adding these targeted PowerFlexes to your routine will add muscle to your arms very quickly. See and feel your muscles as they work, and see the results of them gaining the strength, size, and shape you're seeking. That it your doing a fantastic job, and it shows!

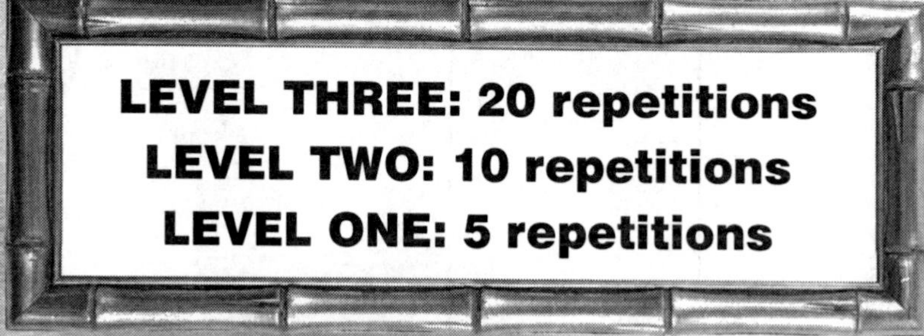

LEVEL THREE: 20 repetitions
LEVEL TWO: 10 repetitions
LEVEL ONE: 5 repetitions

FIGURE 1

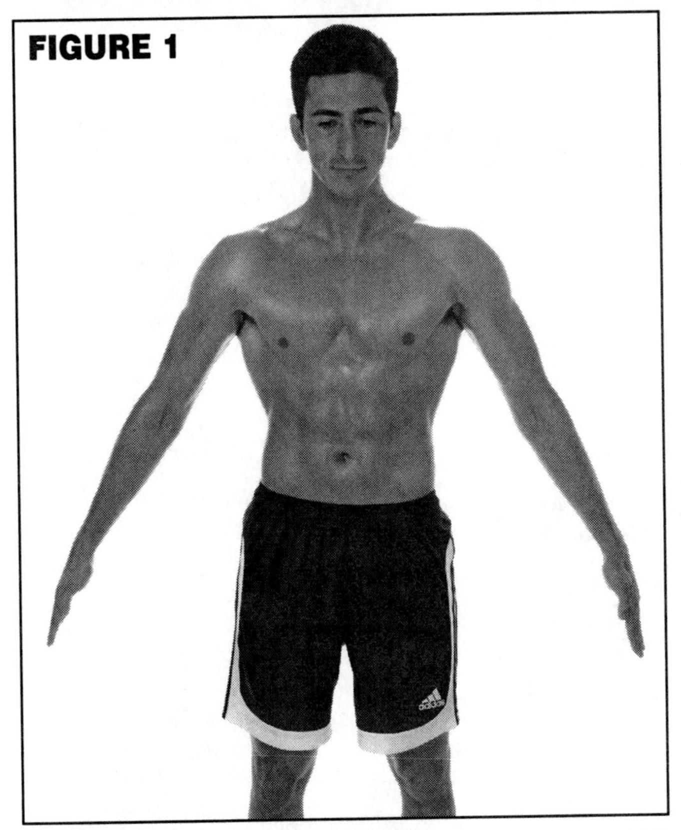

FIGURE 2

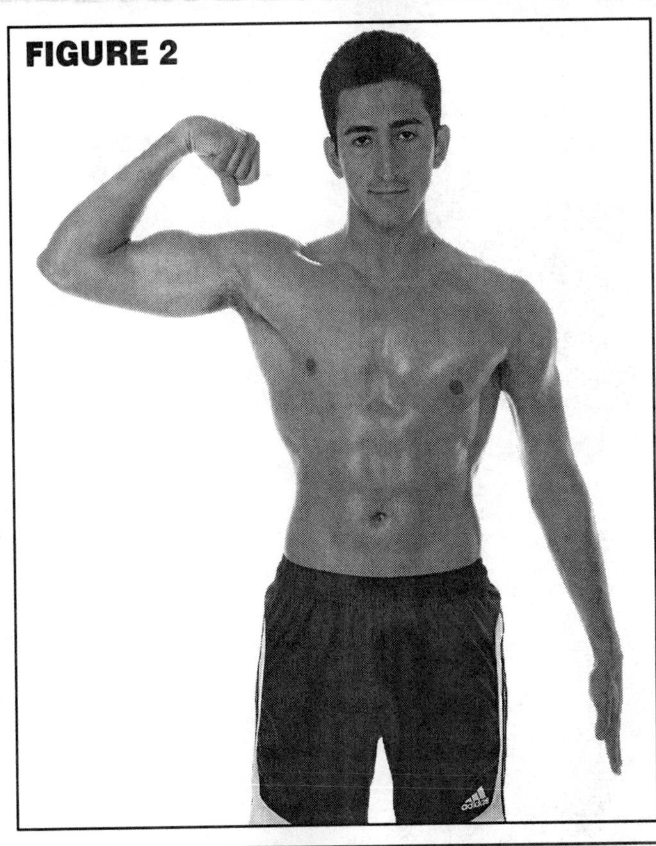

FIGURE 3

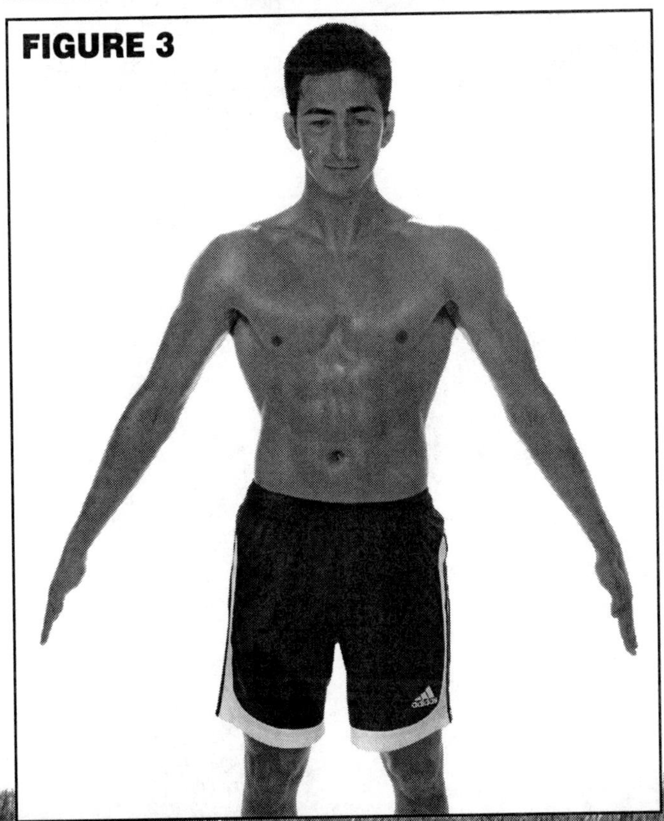

FIGURE 4

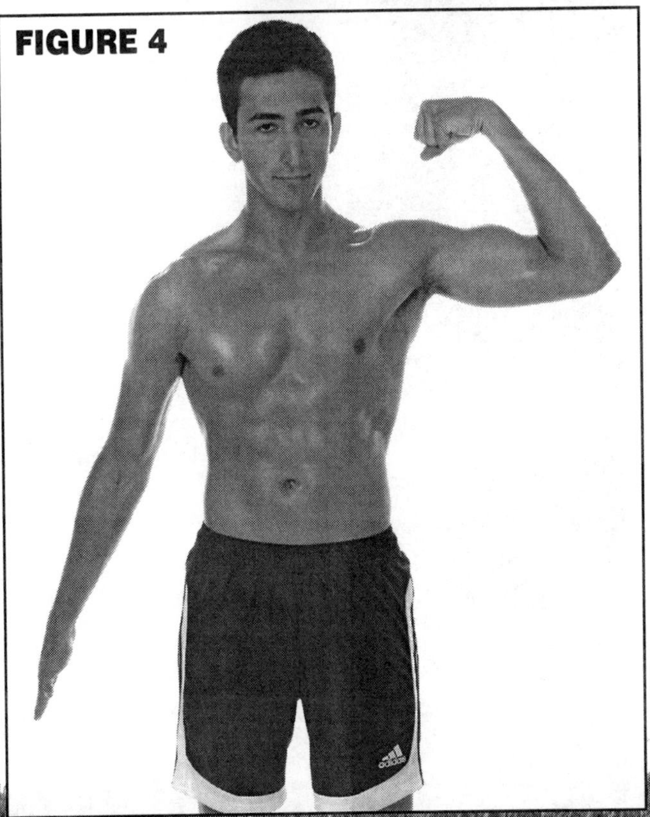

Arm Exercises

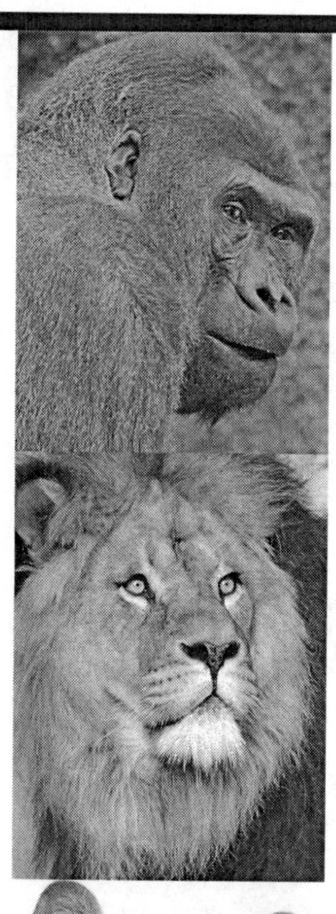

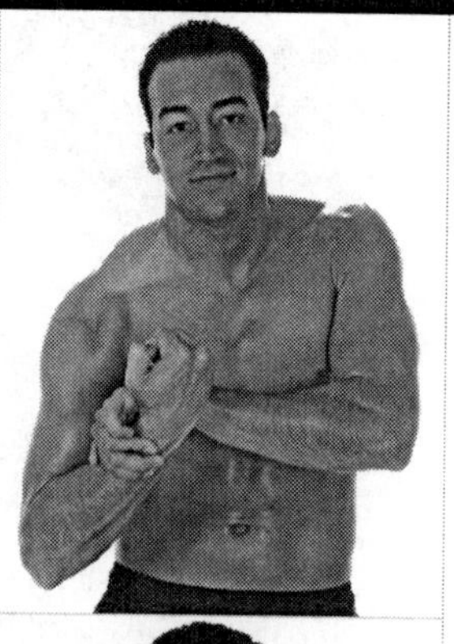

GORILLA FLEX IV

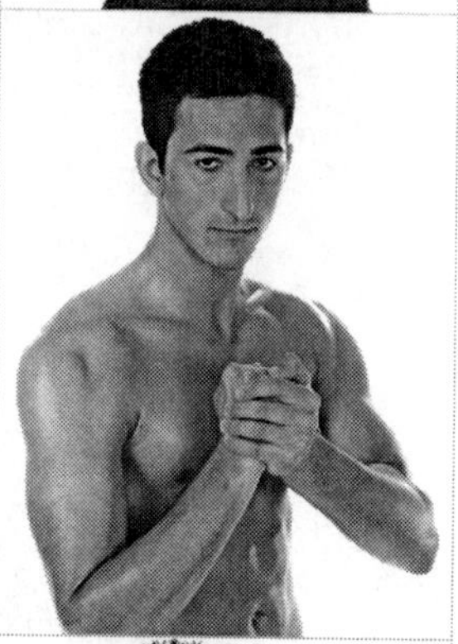

LION FLEX I

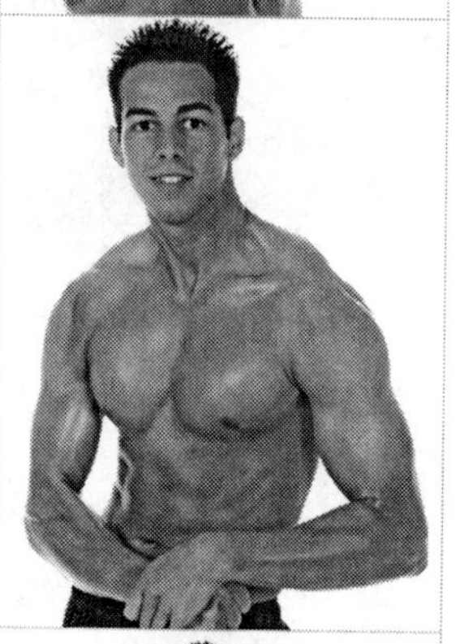

TIGER FLEX I

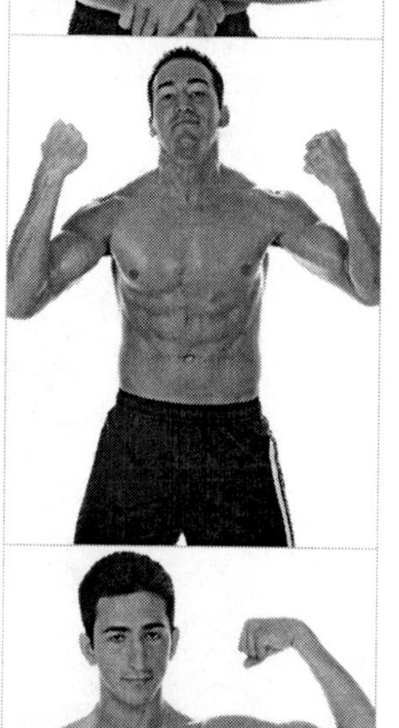

JAGUAR FLEX I

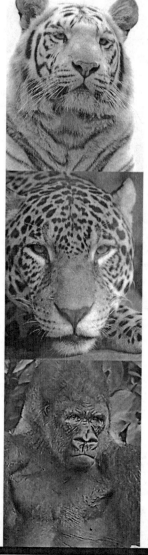

GORILLA FLEX V

POWERFLEX

Speed, Energy & Endurance

SPEED, ENERGY & ENDURANCE WORKOUT

You can have speed, energy, and endurance without using equipment, weights, pulleys, or machines. Just do five PowerFlexes for 20 minutes a day.

Wild Workout® for Speed, Energy, and Endurance

To have a bulging muscular chest, with rippling abs, combined with a healthy flexible spine and firm neck, along with a strong healthy back, powerful attractive well developed legs, well rounded powerful shoulders, combined with muscular strong arms is truly quite an attractive and amazing sight to behold or possess. What really makes a body like this stand out, remarkable, and the cream of the crop is to actually have a lot more than just 'show'. A beautiful body that is actually capable of performing, and is all truly on the inside what it looks like on the outside is awesome! In the animal world you will notice they truly do possess the strength, power, and capabilities on the inside as what it looks like they should from the outside! They are not just all "show" and no "go" but they are all "Show" and all "Go." For instance the eagle can fly to great heights and its powerful talons can snatch huge prey from off the side of a tree, while yet continuing in flight! You're not going to mess with a panther, gorilla, elk, or God forbid a grizzly bear because they will maul you and tear you to ribbons. They do possess the strength on the inside as it looks like they should from the outside.

This is where the Wild Workout® for Speed, Energy, and Endurance steps in. These PowerFlexes are for you to actually attain speed, energy, and endurance which is a real inward capability so your outward body can perform. Theses PowerFlexes bring in the attributes of the cheetah, elk, and the camel. So let's get WILD!

#1—CHEETAH FLEX I

You'll notice the cheetah has a habit of grabbing the grass and dirt with the front paws and pulling back and stretching. Any member of the cat family has that habit, anyone with a housecat know all too well that the couch ends up shredded along with wooden kitchen chair legs, and anything a cat can stick its claws into and stretch. It's the stretching of the muscles that make them durable, able to perform, fills them with stamina and endurance which keeps them from stiffening up and cramping.

Stand with your feet shoulder-width apart and your hands on your hips. Keeping your legs straight, bend forward slowly and smoothly as far as you can without straining. With your right hand, try to touch the floor in front of your left foot. Return to the starting position, then bend forward again. With your left hand, try to touch the floor in front of your right foot. Return to the starting position and repeat.

Don't worry if you can't touch the floor at first, or even your ankle. If you don't feel comfortable reaching below your knee, that's fine—start where you are. Practice this PowerFlex® with consistency and determination and see how quickly your flexibility and endurance improve.

LEVEL THREE: 100 reps (50 per side)
LEVEL TWO: 50 repetitions
LEVEL ONE: 30 repetitions

FIGURE 1

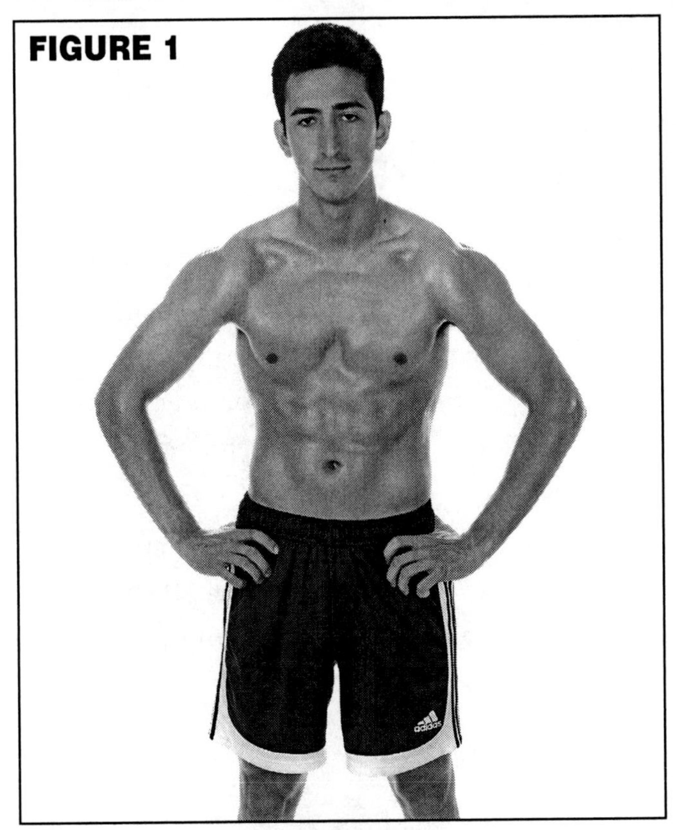

FIGURE 2

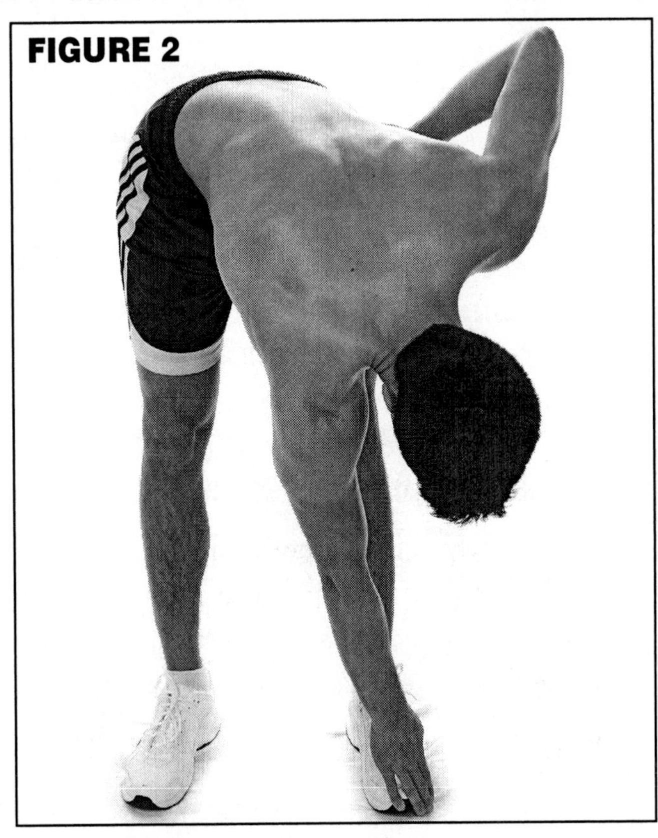

FIGURE 3

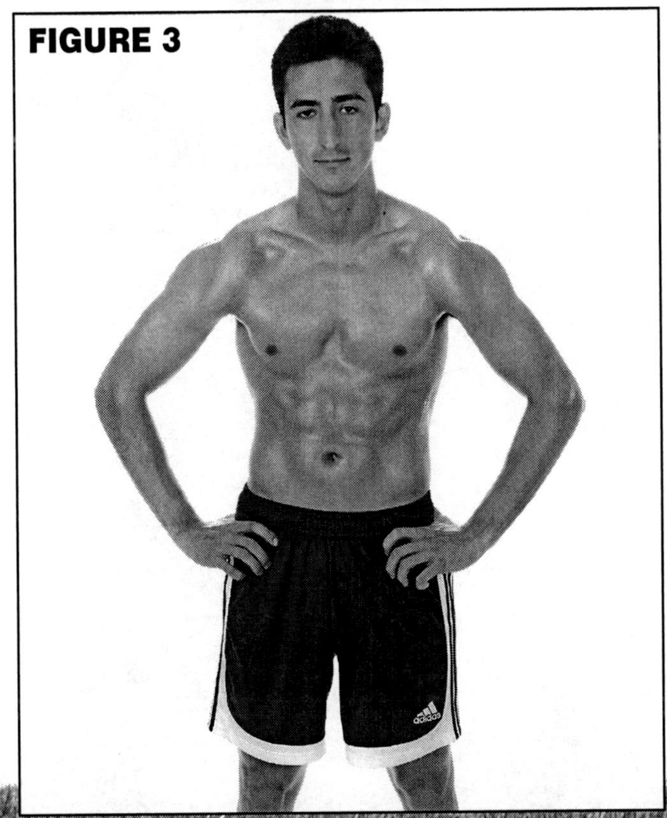

FIGURE 4

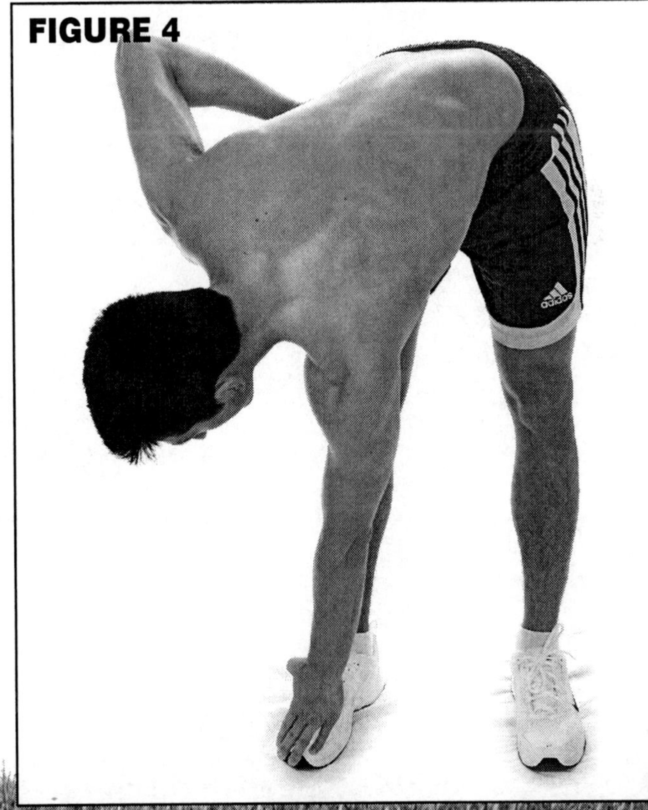

#2—ELK CLIMB

I love to spend time in the high mountains, where the thin air forces some visitors to pant, even when they're standing still. Thanks to Wild Workout®, I have the strength, energy, and endurance to hike and climb at high altitudes. I feel blessed that I can climb high enough to see and appreciate sights people can't see from their cars—such as a half-ton bull elk bounding up a steep slope at 10,000 feet as easily as I'd walk through the meadow far below.

Fortunately, you don't need a mountain to build the fitness to climb one. Just find some stairs. A set of stadium steps or the stairs at an office or apartment building would be ideal, but you can get the same results climbing the stairs in your home. Once you've found some stairs, run up and down them if you can, but if that's a strain, it's fine to walk. This PowerFlex® will build your agility and endurance quickly. One trip up and down counts as one repetition.

LEVEL THREE: 20 repetitions
LEVEL TWO: 10 repetitions
LEVEL ONE: 5 repetitions

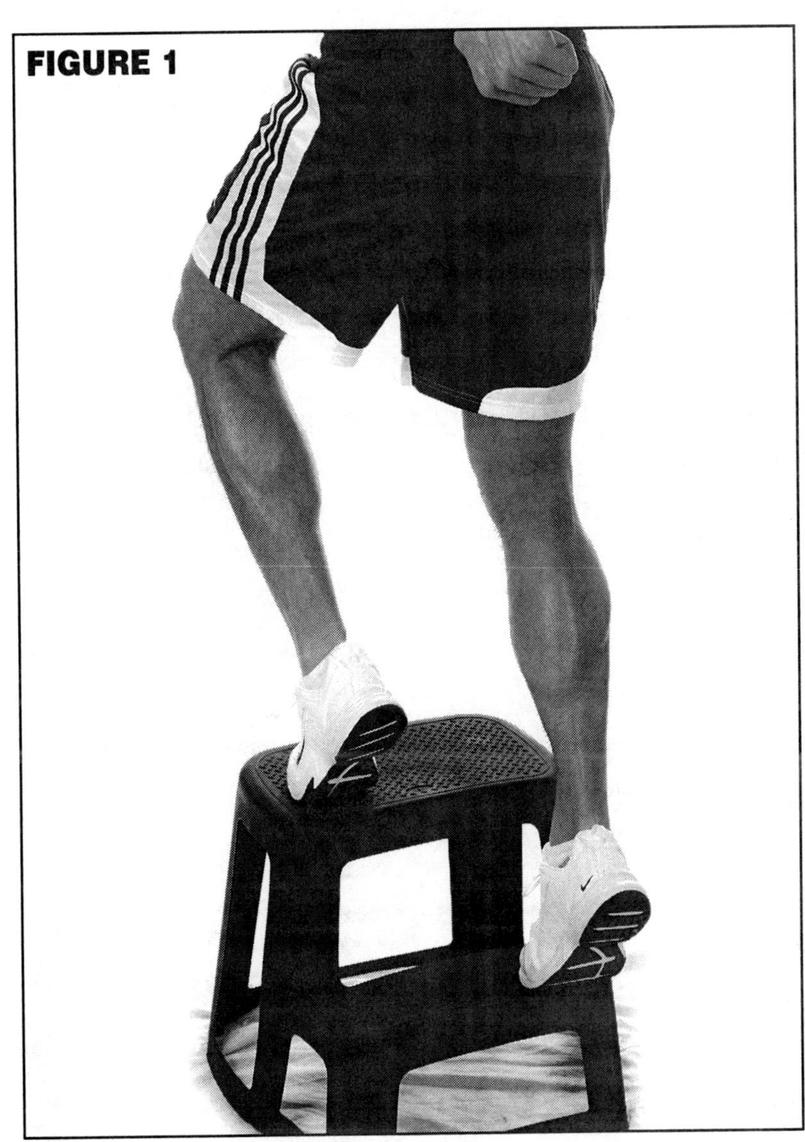
FIGURE 1

#3—CHEETAH DASH

The cheetah is the fastest animal alive on the planet, can reach speeds of 67 miles per hour and over in just 3 seconds flat. It has a burst of speed that makes it fast as grease lightning. No other animal is a match for such blazing speed. The cheetah has amazing speed but it does not run at top speed for a really long distance, about couple hundred yards and that's it. If you're an athlete, you know that winning often depends on speed. It's the difference between getting the takedown and being taken down by your opponent. The difference between catching the touchdown pass and watching it sail through the end zone, just beyond your reach.

First, pace off and mark a 40-yard stretch of grass (at a park or schoolyard or on your own lawn) or track (at a school athletic field) or pavement (on a lightly-traveled street or sidewalk). Now, sprint the distance. Start off with a burst and pump your arms, and don't let up until you've run through your finish line. Rest for 15 seconds (either timed with a stopwatch or counted to yourself), then sprint back to your starting point. Even if you're not an athlete, a burst of speed always comes in handy and it can help you look better too. Research has shown that sprinting not only burns fat more effectively than long distance running but that it builds muscle, too.

Feel free to rest for more than 15 seconds between repetitions, if you need to. In time, you won't need so much rest. Don't strain! If you cannot sprint, that's okay—fast walking works just fine. And you don't need grass, track, or pavement—a large room will do.

LEVEL THREE: 10 repetitions
LEVEL TWO: 7 repetitions
LEVEL ONE: 5 repetitions

FIGURE 1

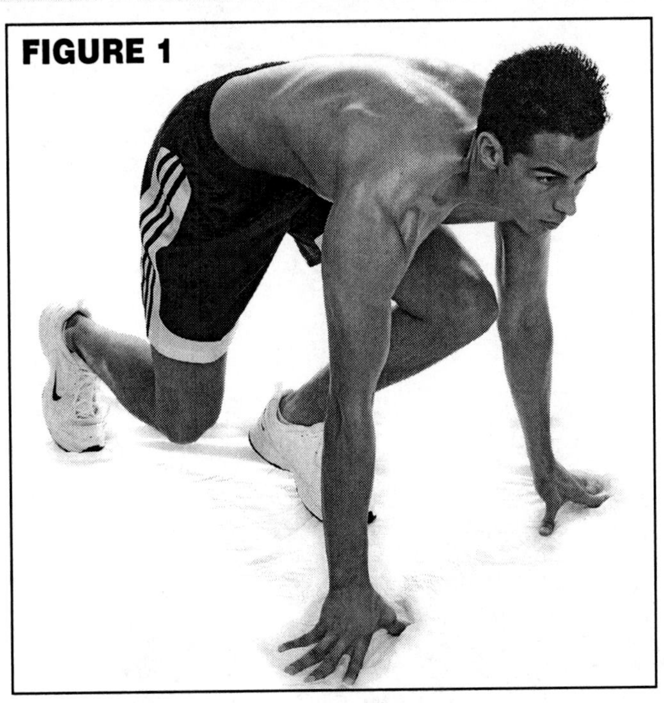

FIGURE 2

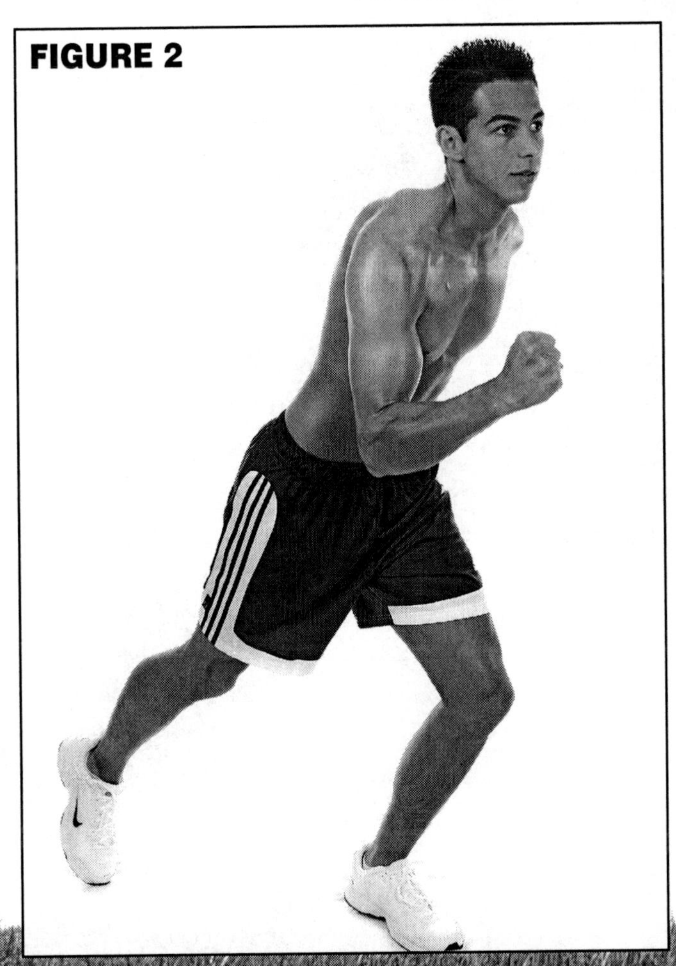

FIGURE 3

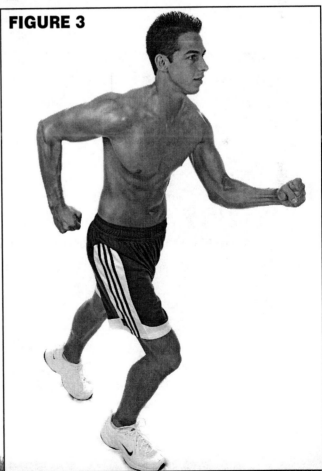

#4—CAMEL TROT

Imagine that a cheetah and a camel decide to run a 200-mile race through the desert. The cheetah will probably jump to a quick lead. But long after the cheetah will have given up, worn out by the distance and the heat, the camel will still be striding slowly and steadily—almost rolling—over the sand to victory. The moral of the story: speed is a valuable trait, whether you're an animal or an athlete. But for complete health and fitness, a human needs endurance, too. That is where the Camel comes in! It might not be the prettiest beast in the world but when it comes to endurance it has it all. It can go on and on for days through the hot scorching desert without even stopping to take a drink. It doesn't blaze through at the speed of a cheetah but long after the cheetah would have been worn out, exhausted, and done in by the heat the camel would still being enduring and going on hot blazing sands, not going fast like a race horse but going long distances at a steady pace. This is the principal of the Camel Trot.

First, measure out a one-mile stretch of grass, track, or sidewalk. If you ran the Cheetah Dash on an outdoor track, you can Camel Trot there, too—a mile equals about four laps. Then, slowly and smoothly jog the distance. The object isn't to break the four-minute mile, but to maintain a slow, steady rhythm. Try to jog like the camel: roll your feet along heel-to-toe instead of slapping them down. Pounding the ground wastes energy and can cause injuries; you will notice the fitness shoes are based upon our principal of the Camel trot rolling heel to toe.

If you're not into competition and you're not out to win any trophies but you just want to be fit and toned with healthy energy and endurance to look and feel great you will want to do this PowerFlex®, but instead of jogging do it as a brisk walk. Walk the distance as briskly as you can the result will be pleasing. Brisk walking is a healing, energizing activity—that's why doctors recommend it so highly, even for heart patients. For humans, walking is the most natural exercise there is. Give yourself the chance to move. And to enjoy moving!

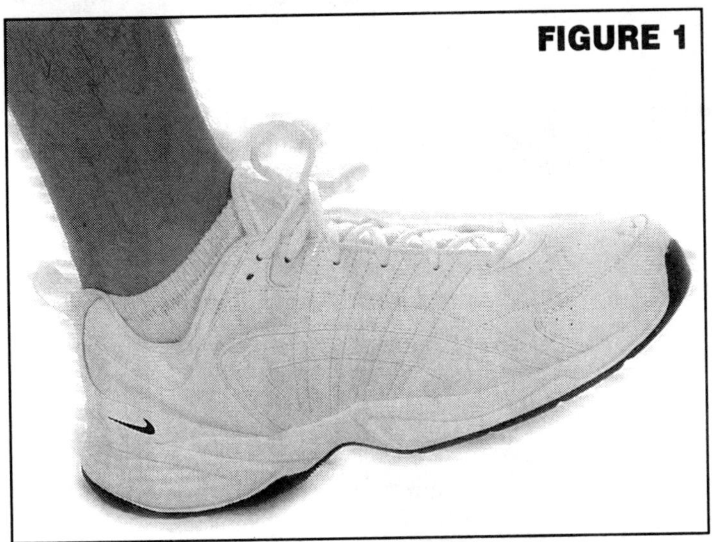
FIGURE 1

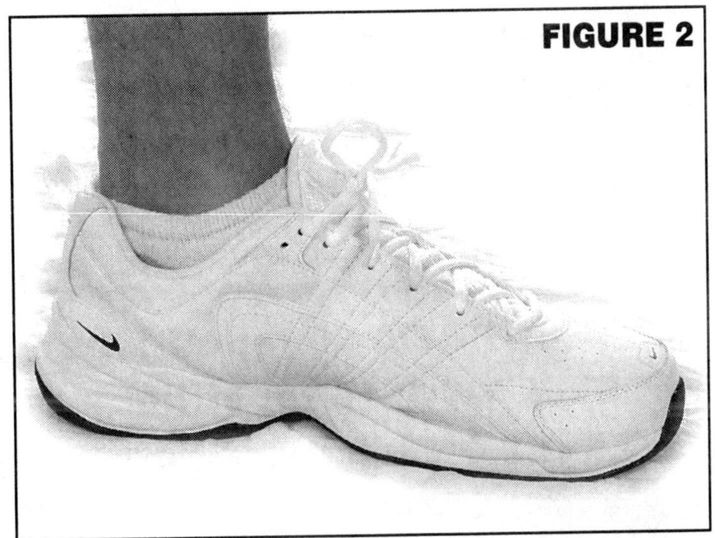
FIGURE 2

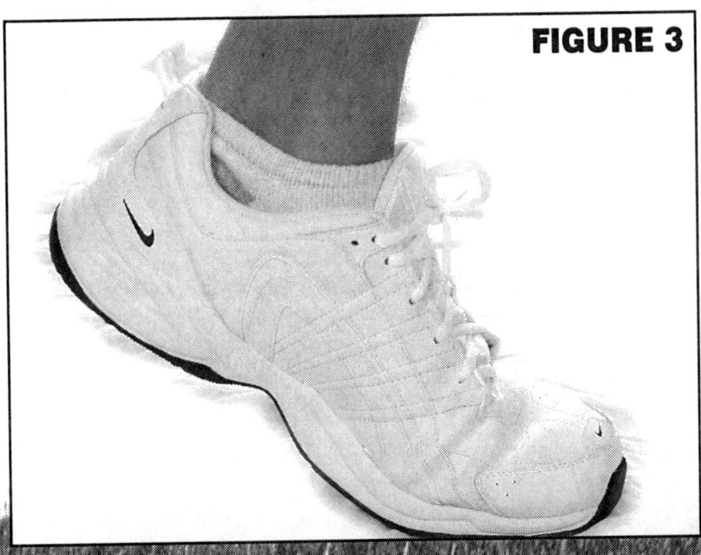
FIGURE 3

#5—CHEETAH FLEX II

Now that you've climbed, dashed, and trotted, your muscles and joints are well warmed up. This last PowerFlex® is similar to Cheetah Flex I and will stretch your legs, hips, and back to help prevent post-workout stiffness and cramping.

Stand with your feet together and your hands on your hips. Keeping your legs straight, bend forward slowly and smoothly as far as you can without straining. With both hands, try to touch the floor in front of your feet. Return to the starting position and repeat.

Don't worry if you can't reach your feet, or even your ankles. Don't bend over farther than you can comfortably. In time, your flexibility will improve; remember it's supposed to feel good!

There you go, friend—the last PowerFlex® in this Wild Workout® course. Practice it with consistency, determination, and patience, and feel the new "Go" your no longer all just "Show."

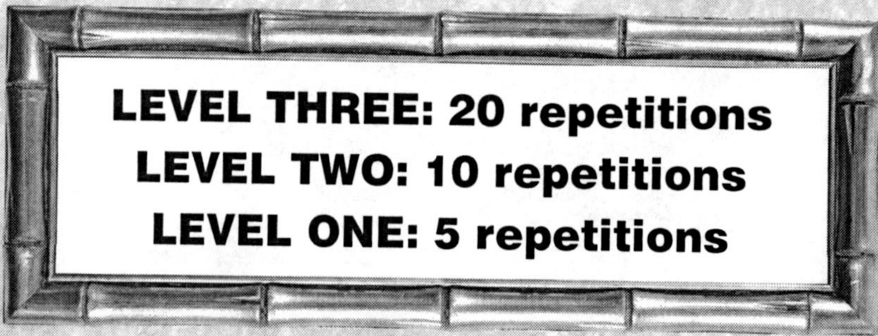

LEVEL THREE: 20 repetitions
LEVEL TWO: 10 repetitions
LEVEL ONE: 5 repetitions

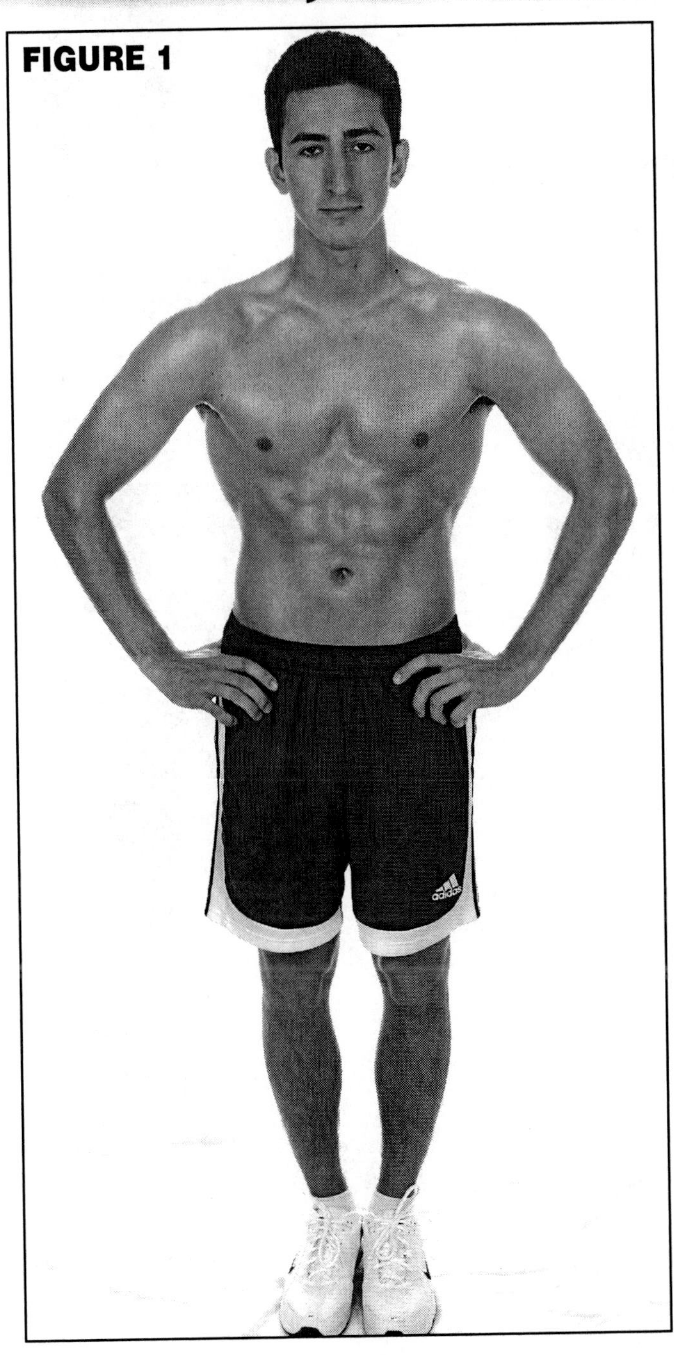

FIGURE 1

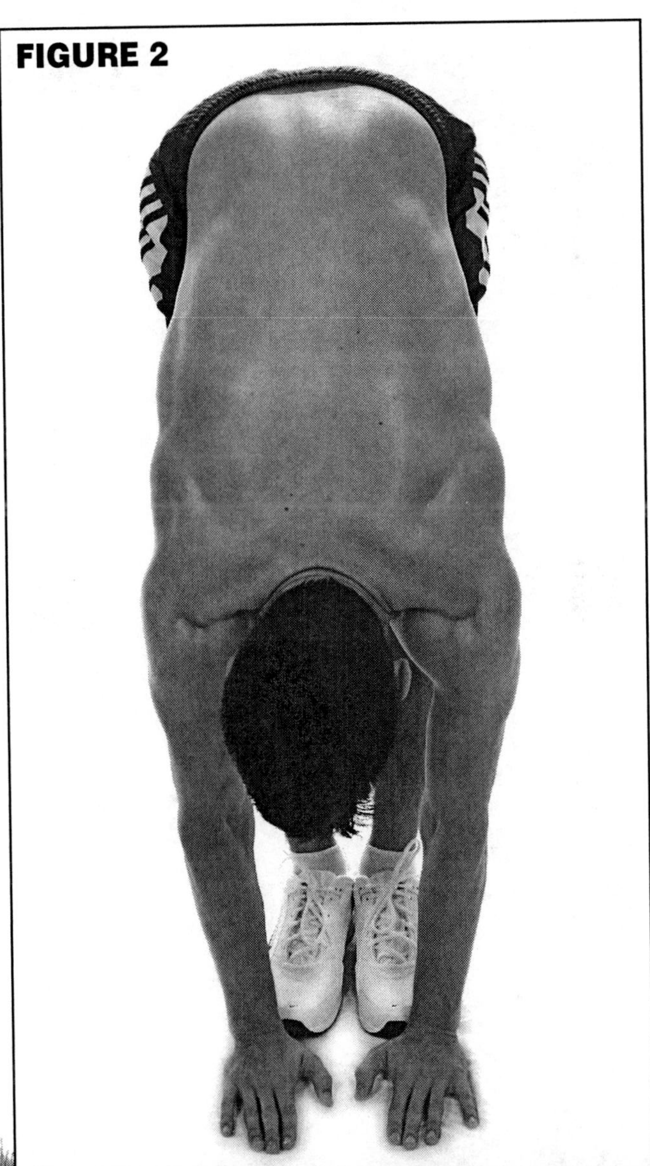
FIGURE 2

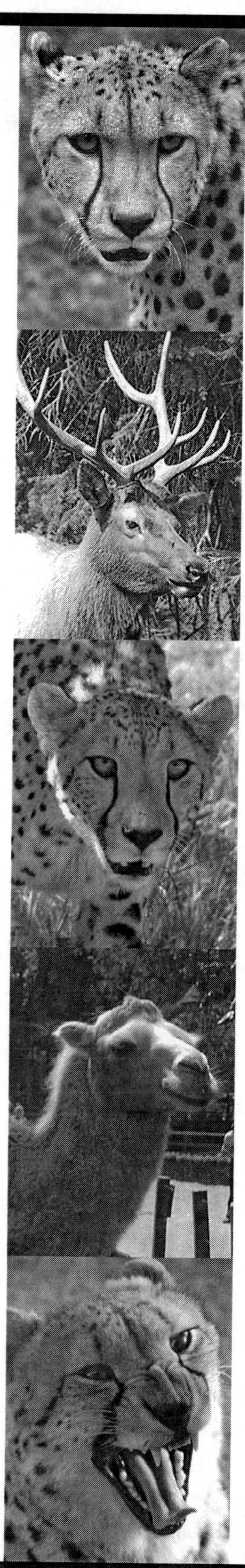

Speed, Energy & Endurance Exercises

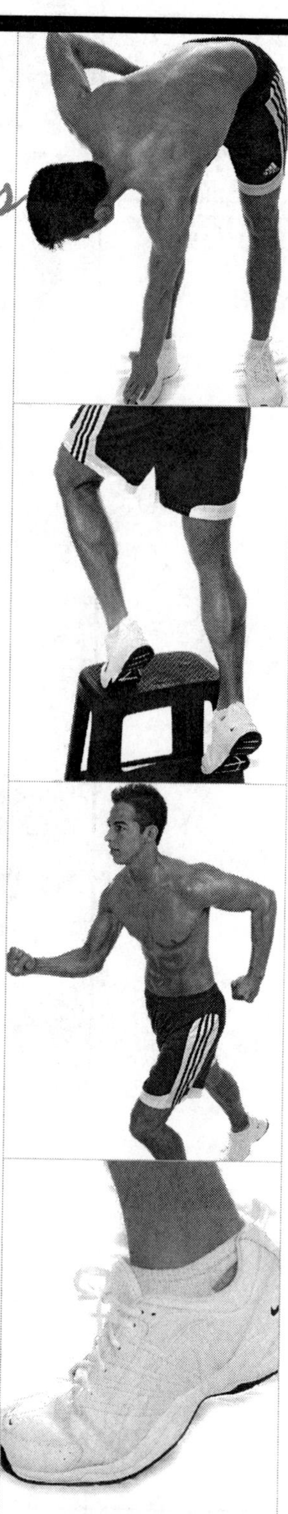

CHEETAH FLEX I

ELK CLIMB

CHEETAH DASH

CAMEL TROT

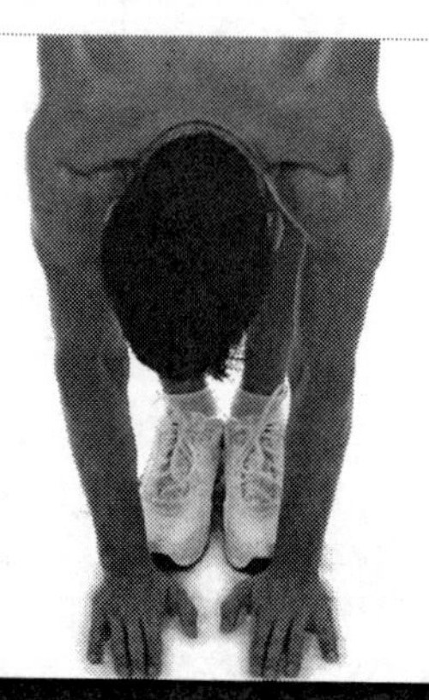

CHEETAH FLEX II

WRAP UP

Dear Friend,

If you've followed the Workout rotation I recommended earlier in this course, you've been doing the Wild Workout® for eight weeks. During that time, you've learned and practiced 45 PowerFlexes—All without using weights, pulleys, bars, bands, machines, or special equipment. Just like the animals you used your own body's energies and abilities to bend, twist, push, pull, flex, and move to build a brand new you! You've seen and felt what it is to work towards a goal and achieve it, But Ohhh No, you're not done yet, this is a workout for life! Whether you want to be healthy, look good, be a champion, beat out competition, or just want to stay fit. The Wild Workout® is it. Continue on and become your own best personal trainer! The Wild Workout® gives you this knowledge and the PowerFlexes are your tools. Isn't fitness fantastic! Continue on to the end of this book and find the treasures of mix and match routines which will excel you to the next level!

I want you to have a diploma recognizing your achievement—something you can frame and look at to remind yourself of where you've come from, where you are, and where you're going. I hope you'll fill out the application on the Certificate of Achievement page and return it to me. If you like, send me a few words about your experience with Wild Workout®. It would be my privilege to rejoice with you in your success. Thank you for allowing me to share this course with you, and for allowing me to help you begin to build the body—and life—you were always meant to have.

Your Friend,

Jim Forystek

Creator, Wild Workout®

Getting to Know the Forysteks

Jimmy Forystek took an interest in exercise at a young age. He entered a national body building contest and earned a trophy only as a teen-ager. Jimmy started his love for sports as a young boy and took his ability and love for football to the college level where he played 4 years of Division 1-FCS football at Liberty University. Jimmy's final season in 2007 the team won the Big South Championship for the first time in the school's history. During Jimmy's freshman year the Flames' new strength coach, who came from the Seattle Seahawks, put the entire team through a strength and endurance, last man standing test he didn't expect anyone to pass. Out of 63 players, Jimmy was one of only three players left standing who made it through the test. Jimmy played wide receiver and proudly wears his championship ring from the Liberty Flames. Jimmy attended college majoring in Business at Liberty University. He also is a Certified PowerFlex® trainer, Instructor, and Fitness Model. Jimmy is the co-author of the Wild Workout® PowerFlex® which is the workout he used to sculpt, build and shape his physique, and it will always be his exclusive workout of choice!

Jimmy's Favorite Routine:

Chest (Direct Target Level 3)
Abdominals (Direct Target Level 3)
Frog Flex I — Level 3
Kangaroo Flex II — Level 3
Speed, Energy and Endurance (Direct Target Level 3)

John Forystek has accomplished many physical tasks all in which he gives credit to his dedication to the Wild Workout®. John is an International model who has over a decade of experience and has used the PowerFlex® program to achieve and maintain his physique. He also is a professional Drummer who has achieved over 25 Gold medals and has been awarded musician of the year by an instrumental publication. John attributes his drumming dexterity, endurance, coordination and speed to the time he spent working out naturally with this unique PowerFlex® program. He is Certified PowerFlex® personal trainer, Fitness Model, and trophy winning Body Builder. He also is co-author of the Wild Workout®!

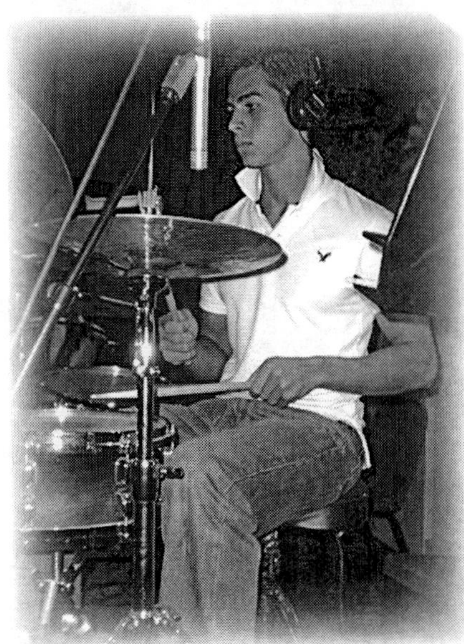

John's Favorite Routine:

100 consecutive Panther Flexes

40 consecutive Bear Flex I

50 consecutive Bull Elk Flex I

60 Dolphin Flex I

100 Dolphin Flex II

40 Gorilla Flex IV

20 Lion Flex I

30 Cougar Flex II

35 Frog Flex I

15 Horse Flex IV

John's After Workout Smoothie:

8 Ice Cubes

1 Cup vanilla yogurt

1 ½ Cups frozen Berries
(I enjoy mixed black berry, raspberries, and blueberries)

2 Cups All-Natural Fruit Juice *(My favorite is a Wild Berry)*

Blend on high until completely mixed

Jed Forystek has a love for tennis and he helped his Tennis team accomplish something they have never done before, which is winning the VIC conference championship for the very first time. Jed has been awarded the Team MVP twice and also the commitment to excellence award for his dedication and example to others in the sport. Jed is also a fitness model, certified PowerFlex® trainer, and co-author of the Wild Workout® which is his personal workout which enhanced his physical abilities allowing him to reach his goals. Jed's college is Liberty University.

Jed's Hard Workout:

100 consecutive panther flexes
60 eagles
40 bears
40 gorillas
40 elks
60 dolphin flex I
100 dolphin flex II
40 shark flex I
100 shark flex II
100 dolphin flex III
100 frog flex I
60 gorilla flex 4
40 frog flex II
60 lion flex I
50 Kangaroo I
60 Tiger I
40 frog III
60 cougar II
60 kangaroo II
60 gorilla III

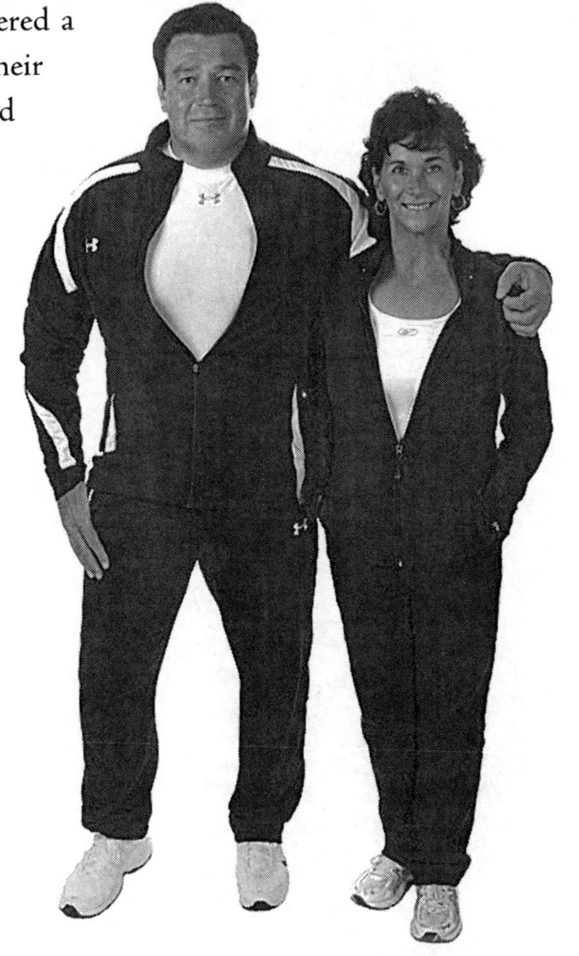

Jim Forystek, Creator of the Wild Workout®, was offered a full college scholarship to be starting full back for their football team by the Chancellor himself. He then Coached and quarterbacked his own city league football team to five championships. Jim has trained teams and individuals to championships in volleyball, soccer, martial arts, bodybuilding, tennis, bowling, track and field and also trains youths to senior citizens on how to get and stay fit so they can enjoy the life that has been given to them. Jim is married to Brenda, a co-fitness enthusiast. Jim is an inspirational and motivational speaker that is in high demand to speak at universities, businesses, churches, trade shows, retreats, assemblies, middle schools, high schools, grade schools, and has appeared on television numerous times as well as on talk radio from the east coast to the west as well as around the world. Jim has appeared in numerous major fitness and muscle magazines as well as newspapers and trade journals across the country. Jim enjoys bringing health and fitness to all people and showing them how easy it can be. If you need a speaker to get your people cranked up on fitness... Jim is the Man!!

How to Easily Reach 100 Panther Flexes:

20 Panther Flexes

20 Eagle Flexes

20 Panther Flexes

20 Bear Flexes

20 Panther Flexes

20 Gorilla Flexes

20 Panther Flexes

20 Elk Flexes

20 Panther Flexes

(Rest as needed between each set)

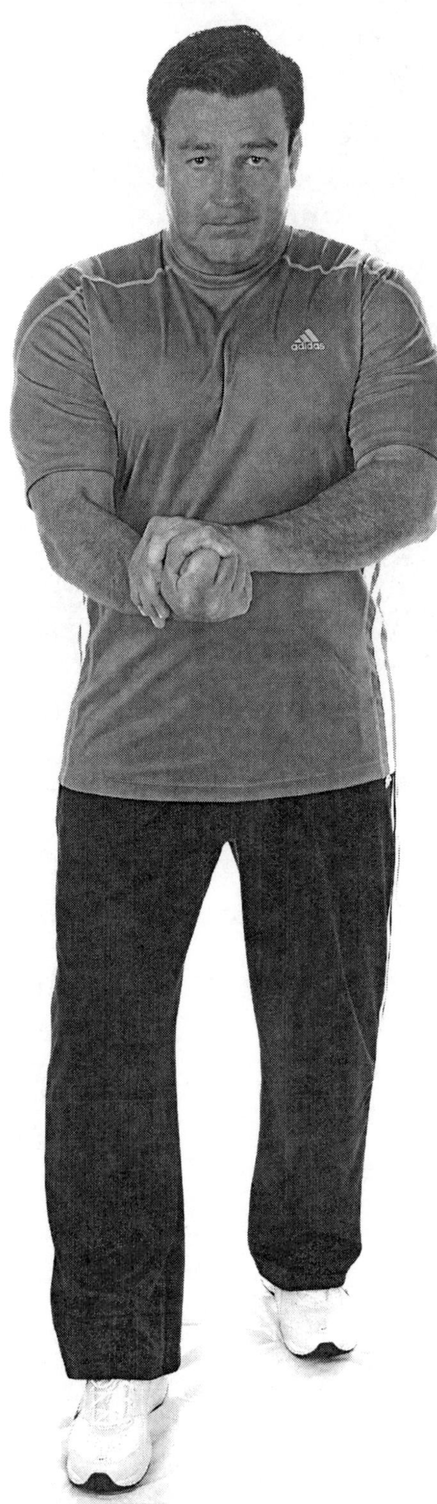

Jim's Favorite Power Snack:

1 Handful of unsalted peanuts

1 Heaping handful of Raw Almonds

1 Peeled orange

1 bottle of pure artesian drinking water

WILDWORKOUT® POWERFLEX® ROUTINES

Welcome to the WildWorkout® PowerFlex® Routine Section. Here you will learn all about our WildWorkout® Routines. Starting with finding exactly what you are looking to accomplish, we'll show you how to arrive at the routine, and you can either pick from a pre-made routine, find a routine where you can add the exercises or your choice or use our approaches and routines to help build the perfect routine for yourself as we help you to become your own best personal trainer with WildWorkout®. We understand that each person is a unique individual with different personalities, likes, dislikes, body-types, shapes, desires and goals. Here you will find many different structured routines that will get you great results, and is exactly what you are looking for. We will also show you how to structure you own personal routines to help you become YOUR OWN BEST PERSONAL TRAINER! You will never have to get bored of doing the same old routine over and over again! Whether you want to mix up your workout every 8 weeks, 4 weeks, weekly, or even daily with WildWorkout® PowerFlex® we will show you how!

There are three main approaches to consider when choosing or structuring your routines. Whether you are a beginner and this is your first time ever exercising, or whether you are an avid exerciser, you can use these three routine approaches to get exactly what you want out of exercising. Whether you use each individual approach, put two together, or use all three together to have an exciting, fun WildWorkout® PowerFlex® routine you love!

Before you start choosing and structuring your workout you must decide WHAT IS YOUR GOAL/ TARGET! It can be simple and very basic or go as detailed as you want. You can have a simple goal of you want to lose 10 pounds and get definition in your abs, or you can go more detailed and want six-pack abs while getting a full body workout, maintaining big pecs, and getting a lot of cardio. You can decide if you want to start an 8 week routine, or just do daily routines. Define your goals whether big or small, basic or detailed. It could also be just listing your problem areas are and what you want to improve. Do you want to get lean, sculpted and ripped? Do you want strong, huge bulging muscles? Or are you just looking for a basic workout to keep you healthy? When it comes to WildWorkout® PowerFlex®, through our help, YOU CAN BECOME YOUR OWN BEST PERSONAL TRAINER! After all, YOU know YOURSELF the best! Decide what you want and find the routine that best suites you and that you feel will best help you achieve your goals, or use these approaches and routines to help develop your own custom WildWorkout® PowerFlex® routine. Remember you can start slow and work your way to where you want to be! Being fit & healthy doesn't come overnight in one day, but it's a day by day, week by week, month by month process. The key is to keep consistent week after week and also remember to keep track of what you have done, or haven't done, ate or didn't eat, and write it all in your WildWorkout® PowerFlex® Journal! You cannot eat an entire elephant all in one bite, but it's a bite by bite process that gets the job done. With defining your goals you can start small and work your way bigger, build your confidence and remember becoming and maintaining a fit and healthy lifestyle is not just a one-time thing, but it is a choice that you'll learn to love and something you will want to do regularly because of how much joy and satisfaction you will get from it.

The first approach is the **DIRECT TARGET APPROACH.** In the direct target approach you are going to approach your exercises in full sections, exercise by exercise. If you decide you want to start your path to 6-pack abs, you will take the abdominal section in one workout performing one exercise at a time resting between exercises and sets, concentrating specifically on that exercise until it is complete. Then you will move on to the next exercise. You can break each exercise into sets resting between each set, or do them all in one continuous set and resting between exercises. For example if want to exercise your ABDOMINALS with the Direct Target Approach you will do:

Dolphin Flex 1 (Level 1-3 Until Complete)
Short Rest (30 seconds – 3 Minutes)
Dolphin Flex 2 (Level 1-3 Until Complete)
Short Rest (30 seconds – 3 Minutes)
Shark Flex 1 (Level 1-3 Until Complete)
Short Rest (30 seconds – 3 Minutes)
Shark Flex 2 (Level 1-3 Until Complete)
Short Rest (30 seconds – 3 Minutes)
Dolphin Flex 3 (Level 1-3 Until Complete)

You may perform Level 1-Level 3 Repetitions remembering that Level Three is for optimal performance, satisfaction, and results. Always train and never strain, if you need to start at level one, start at level one. Break each exercise up into sets as well, as you do not need to perform any exercise repetitions all in a row (unless you want to or can). For example if performing the Panther Flex I Level 3 you don't need to do 100 in a row (as many people cannot) but break them into sets. See below

10 Sets of 10 Repetitions in a row (10x10=100)

Rest between each set. (30 sec - 3 min)

5 Sets of 20 Repetitions

4 Sets of 25 Repetitions

2 Sets of 30 Reps & 2 Sets of 20 Reps

2 Sets 50 Reps

Break them down however you feel comfortable

In the Direct Target Approach you may also be specifically targeting more than one muscle group in a single workout. For example you could want to work your Arms, Shoulders and Back all in one workout in one day. Choose which section of your choices you want to start with and perform that section until complete, move onto the next section, and then the last section doing each section laid out with the abdominal section example above.

The second approach is the **MIX AND MATCH APPROACH**. In the mix and match approach you are going to approach your exercises by mixing and matching them into your routine to give you a creative, fun way to put your exercises together to get a great workout. In the Mix and Match Approach you do not have to perform the entire section like with the Direct Target Approach (unless you want to). For example if you want to work your abs, chest, arms, back and legs all in one workout in one day, you may not have the time using the Direct Target Approach, but with the Mix and Match approach you can choose 1-3 exercises from each section you are looking to work and put them together for a creative, unique workout routine that could look something like this.

Dolphin Flex 1 (Level 1-3 Until Complete)

Short Rest

Shark Flex 2 (Level 1-3 Until Complete)

Short Rest

Panther Flex 1 (Level 1-3 Until Complete)

Short Rest

Eagle Flex 1 (Level 1-3 Until Complete)

Short Rest

Gorilla Flex IV (Level 1-3 Until Complete)

Short Rest

Lion Flex I (Level 1-3 Until Complete)

Short Rest

Horse Flex I (Level 1-3 Until Complete)

Short Rest

Mule Flex (Level 1-3 Until Complete)

Short Rest

Frog Flex I (Level 1-3 Until Complete)

Short Rest

Frog Flex II (Level 1-3 Until Complete)

In this example you are performing 10 exercises from five different sections which would be about the same workout time as performing two sections from the Direct Target Approach.

How to use The Mix and Match Approach and the Direct Target Approach at the same time: You can easily put the Direct Target Approach and the Mix and Match Approach together in one workout by Directly Targeting one or two sections and mix and matching a couple other sections. You could directly target the Abs and Arms, while Mix and Matching the Chest, Legs, and Neck.

The Third Approach is the **CIRCUIT APPROACH.** In the Circuit Approach you are going to approach your exercises by doing them in a continuous circuit. This approach is not only great for muscle building but also fantastic for fat burning! On days where you are looking for a great cardio workout and don't quite feel like doing the Speed, Energy and Endurance section and putting your running shoes on, do the Circuit Approach! In the Circuit Approach you will be performing one exercise right after another with no rest time in between. In this approach you will only perform one set of a particular exercise then move to the next exercise set and when you've completed one set of each of all desired exercises you will come back to the beginning and perform each exercise set again until you reach your desired number of repetitions for those exercises. There are multiple approaches to the Circuit approach and you can find the one you enjoy the best.

For example if you want to perform the Chest and Abdominal sections (full sections like in the Direct Target Approach) you could do so using the Circuit Approach. You can do both sections, all 10 exercises in a single circuit, or do each section by itself in a circuit (5 exercises at a time) or pair them two by two.

If performing both exercises in one circuit, have a starting number that's easily obtainable for at least 2 times through the circuit. So let's say you are going to start performing each exercise for 10 repetitions. You will perform the following with NO REST. Once you complete the circuit once then you can have a short rest if you must before performing it again. (Of course if you have to rest during the circuit you can, just try to set your reps at a reasonable number where you will not tire yourself out too quickly). If performing two sections together in a single circuit try alternating each exercise from one section then the next section to give your muscle groups a rest so you will not tire out one muscle group too fast.

Panther Flex I — 10 Reps
Dolphin Flex I — 10 Reps
Eagle Flex I — 10 Reps
Dolphin Flex II — 10 Reps
Bear Flex I — 10 Reps
Shark Flex I — 10 Reps
Gorilla Flex I — 10 Reps
Shark Flex II — 10 Reps
Elk Flex I — 10 Reps
Dolphin Flex III — 10 Reps
(Repeat with no rest between exercises until desired level is reached)

A good goal to set is performing through each circuit at least 3 times.

If you wanted to pair exercises in twos until finished you could do it this way:

Panther Flex I — 10 Reps
Dolphin Flex I — 10 Reps
(Repeat until exercise level complete)
Eagle Flex I — 10 Reps

Dolphin Flex II — 10 Reps
(Repeat until exercise level complete)
ETC...

Using the Circuit Approach is also great with the Mix and Match Approach. You can use multiple circuits or just one. You could Mix and Match Chest, Abs, Legs, & Back choosing 1 exercise from each and putting them into a circuit that could look like this:

Panther Flex I — 15 Reps
No Rest
Dolphin Flex I — 10 Reps
No Rest
Frog Flex I — 20 Reps
No Rest
Horse Flex I — 5 Reps
(Perform Circuit 5 Times)

All the reps do not have to be the same for each exercise. Some exercises you may be better at performing, and some you may need improvement. You can have a higher or lower number of reps for each exercise, and use them for your circuit. The exercises themselves do not need to be performed speedily in the Circuit Approach; but make sure there is no rest time between exercises unless absolutely necessary.

Daily, Weekly & Group Routines

During the WildWorkout® PowerFlex® Routines remember to drink water before, during and after workouts. If you ever get exhausted stop, rest and drink water. Start slow and work your way up. It is advised you start with the introductory eight week program to learn all 45 different exercises and build a good foundational strength and physique for you to continue to build upon with the WildWorkout® PowerFlex® Routines. We recommend you workout 3-5 days per week. The following routines have daily routines in which you can pick from day to day workouts finding what routine you feel like doing that day, weekly routines, 4 week routines, and 8 week routines. Depending on your schedule, family, work, meetings, etc., we expect your exercise schedule to work around you, not you around it. With WildWorkout® PowerFlex® You don't have to drive to the gym, you don't have to have to schedule an appointment, but you can exercise in the privacy of your own home, backyard, hotel, park, basement, garage, wherever you are, when it's convenient for YOU!

When you a section listed with (Direct Target) following the section means you will do that entire section (5 exercises) via the Direct Target Approach. When you see a section listed with (Mix & Match Pick One, Two or Three) it means to pick as many exercises from that section as listed. If you see a routine listed as a Circuit Routine, use the Circuit routine approach remembering that no rest is supposed to be used between exercises.

DAILY ROUTINE

Approach: Direct Target

Concentration: Chest, Abs, Arms

Chest (Direct Target)

Abs (Direct Target)

Arms (Direct Target)

DAILY ROUTINE

Approach: Direct Target

Concentration: Legs, Abs, Speed, Energy & Endurance

Legs (Direct Target)

Abs (Direct Target)

Speed, Energy & Endurance (Direct Target)

DAILY ROUTINE

Approach: Direct Target and Mix & Match

Concentration: Chest & Back (Direct Target); Legs, Arms, Abs (Mix & Match)

Chest (Direct Target)

Arms (Pick One)

Abs (Pick One)

Back (Direct Target)

Legs (Pick One)

DAILY ROUTINE

Approach: Direct Target and Mix & Match

Concentration: Legs & Abs (Direct Target); Chest & Shoulders (Mix & Match)

Legs (Direct Target)

Chest (Panther Flex I & Pick One)

Abs (Direct Target)

Shoulders (Pick Two)

DAILY ROUTINE

Approach: Direct Target and Mix & Match

Concentration: Arms & Abs (Direct Target); Chest & Legs (Mix & Match)

Arms (Direct Target)

Chest (Panther Flex I & Pick One)

Abs (Direct Target)

Legs (Pick Two)

DAILY ROUTINE

Approach: Mix & Match

Concentration: Chest, Abs, Back, Speed, Energy & Endurance

Chest (Panther Flex I & Pick One)

Abs (Dolphin Flex I & Pick One)

Back (Horse Flex I & Pick One)

Speed, Energy & Endurance (Elk Climb & Pick One)

DAILY ROUTINE

Approach: Mix & Match

Concentration: Chest, Shoulders, Neck, Speed, Energy & Endurance

Chest (Panther Flex I & Pick One)

Shoulders (Pick Three)

Neck (Pick Three)

Speed, Energy and Endurance (Camel Trot & Pick One)

DAILY ROUTINE

FULL BODY POWER WORKOUT

Approach: Direct Target and Mix & Match

Chest (Direct Target)

Abdominals (Direct Target)

Legs (Direct Target)

Arms (Mix & Match -Pick Two)

Shoulders (Mix & Match -Pick Two)

Back (Mix & Match -Pick Two)

Neck (Mix & Match -Pick Two)

Spine (Mix & Match -Pick Two)

Speed, Energy, & Endurance (Direct Target)

DAILY ROUTINE

FAT BURNING, MUSCLE SCULPTING, DOUBLE CIRCUIT

Approach: Circuit

Concentration: Full Body

Chest- Panther Flex I- 10 Reps

Legs - Frog Flex I - 10 Reps

Abs- Dolphin Flex I- 10 Reps

Chest- Eagle Flex I – 5 Reps

Legs- Kangaroo Flex II – 6 Reps (per leg)

Abs- Shark Flex II – 5 Reps (each way)

(Perform Circuit 3-6 Times)

(Short Rest & Water)

Speed, Energy and Endurance - Elk Climb- 5 Reps

Shoulders- Gorilla Flex II – 10 Reps (each arm)

Back- Horse Flex IV - 5 Reps

Arms- Jaguar Flex I – 5 Reps

Speed, Energy and Endurance- Cheetah Flex I- 5 Reps (per side)

Shoulders- Cougar Flex II - 5 Reps (each arm)

Back- Horse Flex I - 5 Reps (each side)

Arms- Tiger Flex I – 5 Reps (each arm)

(Perform Circuit 2-4 Times)

DAILY ROUTINE

QUICK STRENGTHENING – TIME CRUNCH CIRCUIT

Approach: Circuit

Concentration: Chest, Abs, Legs

Chest- Panther Flex I - 10 Reps

Abs- Dolphin Flex I - 10 Reps

Legs - Frog Flex I - 10 Reps

Abs- Dolphin Flex II - 10 Reps

(Perform Circuit 3-6 times)

WEEKLY ALTERNATE DAY ROUTINE

Approach Used: Direct Target and Mix & Match

Chest, Abs, Legs, & Back (Direct Targets)

Your Choice (Mix & Match)

Speed, Energy and Endurance (Mix & Match)

Day 1: Chest & Abs (Direct Target)

- Mix & Match Pick 3
- Elk Climb & Camel Trot

Day 2: Legs & Back (Direct Target)

- Mix & Match Pick 3

Camel Trot & Cheetah Dash

(Repeat for days 3-6 Rest Day 7)

3-DAY WEEKLY POWER ROUTINE

Sunday-Tuesday-Thursday

Approach: Direct Target and Mix & Match

Concentration: Chest, Abs, Speed Energy & Endurance (Direct Target)

Full Body (Mix & Match)

Chest (Direct Target)

Abs (Direct Target)

Arms (Mix & Match -Pick Two)

Shoulders (Mix & Match -Pick Two)

Legs (Mix & Match -Frog Flex I + Pick One)

Neck, Spine, Back (Mix & Match -Pick One)

Speed, Energy and Endurance (Direct Target)

4-WEEK ABS & CARDIO BLASTER WILDWORKOUT® ROUTINE

Approach: Direct Target, Mix & Match, and Circuit

Concentration: Abdominals & Cardiovascular

Level: Your Choice

WEEK 1

Day 1 & Day 4: Abs (Direct Target), Circuit: Panther Flex I - 15 Reps, Frog Flex I - 15 Reps, Mule Flex - 5 Reps (Perform Circuit 4 Times), Speed, Energy & Endurance (Direct Target)

Day 2 & Day 5: Circuit: Dolphin Flex I, Dolphin Flex II, Shark Flex I, Shark Flex II, Dolphin Flex III (Perform Circuit 3-5 Times), Speed, Energy & Endurance (Direct Target)

Day 3, Day 6, & Day 7: Off (Feel free to rest, or use a desired daily routine)

WEEK 2

Day 1 & Day 4: Circuit: Dolphin Flex I 10-15 Reps, Panther Flex I 10-20 Reps, Dolphin

Flex II 15-25 Reps, Frog Flex I 10-20 Reps, Shark Flex I 5-15 Reps (Perform Circuit 4-6 Times) Circuit: Shark Flex II 10-20 Reps (Each Way), Elk Climb 4-6 Reps, Dolphin Flex III 15-25 Reps, Mule Flex 5-10 Reps (Perform Circuit 3-5 Times), Camel Trot

Day 2 & Day 5: Abdominals (Direct Target), Circuit: Panther Flex I – 10 Reps, Frog Flex I – 10 Reps, Gorilla Flex I – 5 Reps (Perform Circuit 3-7 Times), Speed, Energy, and Endurance (Direct Target)

Day 3, 6, 7: Off

WEEK 3

Day 1 & Day 4: Camel Trot, Abdominals (Direct Target), Elk Climb

Day 2 & Day 5: Abdominals (Direct Target), Circuit: Panther Flex I – 10 Reps, Frog Flex I – 10 Reps, Elk Flex I – 5 Reps (Each Way) (Perform Circuit 3-7 Times), Speed, Energy, and Endurance (Direct Target)

Day 3, 6, 7: Off

WEEK 4

Day 1 & Day 4: Abdominals (Direct Target (Suggested: Level Three)), Speed, Energy, and Endurance (Direct Target (Suggested: Level Three))

Day 2 & Day 5: Circuit: Dolphin Flex I – 8 Reps, Dolphin Flex II – 12 Reps, Shark Flex I – 5 Reps, Shark Flex II – 10 Reps (5 Each Way), Dolphin Flex III – 12 Reps (Perform Circuit 3 Times) Circuit: Panther Flex I – 15 Reps, Dolphin Flex I – 8 Reps, Dolphin Flex II – 12 Reps, Frog Flex I – 15 Reps, Shark Flex I – 5 Reps, Horse Flex I – 5 Reps, Shark Flex II – 10 Reps (5 Each Way), Dolphin Flex III – 12 Reps, Eagle Flex I – 5 Reps (Perform Circuit 3-5 Times)

Day 3, 6, 7: Off

A 4-WEEK GET FIT, DON'T HOLD BACK WILDWORKOUT® ROUTINE

Approach: Direct Target and Mix & Match

Concentration: Total Body

WEEK 1

Monday & Thursday: Target Muscles → Chest and Abdominal

Panther Flex I – 4 sets of 20 reps; Eagle Flex I – 2 sets of 20 reps; Bear Flex I – 2 sets of 15 reps; Gorilla Flex I – 2 sets of 15 reps; Elk Flex I – 2 sets of 10 reps (5 Each Arm)

Dolphin Flex I – 2 sets of 30 reps; Dolphin Flex II – 3 sets of 30 reps; Shark Flex I – 2 sets of 20 reps; Shark Flex II – 1 set of 20 reps; Dolphin Flex III – 3 sets of 30 reps

Tuesday & Friday: Target Muscles → Legs and Shoulders

Legs: Frog Flex I – 4 sets of 20 reps; Frog Flex II – 2 sets of 10 reps; Kangaroo Flex I – 2 sets of 15 reps; Frog Flex III – 2 sets of 10 reps; Kangaroo Flex II – 3 sets of 5 reps each leg

Shoulders: Gorilla Flex II – 2 sets of 20 reps; Gorilla Flex III – 2 sets of 20 reps; Rhino Flex I – 2 sets of 20 reps; Cougar Flex I – 2 sets of 20 reps; Cougar Flex II – 2 sets of 20 reps

Wednesday & Saturday: Cardiovascular

Elk Climb: 2 sets of 5 reps; Cheetah Dash: 5 reps; Camel Trot: One mile jog

WEEK 2

Monday & Thursday: Target Muscles → Chest and Abdominal

Panther Flex I – 4 sets of 22 reps; Eagle Flex I – 2 sets of 20 reps; Bear Flex I – 2 sets of 15 reps; Gorilla Flex I – 2 sets of 15 reps; Elk Flex I – 2 sets of 10 reps (5 Each Arm)

Dolphin Flex I – 2 sets of 30 reps; Dolphin Flex II – 3 sets of 30 reps; Shark Flex I – 2 sets of 20 reps; Shark Flex II – 1 set of 20 reps; Dolphin Flex III – 3 sets of 30 reps

Tuesday & Friday: Target Muscles → Legs and Arms

Frog Flex I – 4 sets of 20 reps; Frog Flex II – 2 sets of 10 reps; Kangaroo Flex I – 2 sets of 15 reps; Frog Flex III – 2 sets of 10 reps; Kangaroo Flex II – 3 sets of 5 reps each leg

Gorilla Flex IV – 2 sets of 20 reps; Lion Flex I – 2 sets of 20 reps; Tiger Flex I – 2 sets of 10 reps; Jaguar Flex I – 2 sets 10; Gorilla Flex V – 2 sets of 10 reps

Wednesday & Saturday: Cardiovascular

Camel Trot: One mile jog; Elk Climb: 2 sets of 5 reps; Cheetah Dash: 6 reps

WEEK 3

Monday & Thursday: Target Muscles → Chest and Back

Panther Flex I – 4 sets of 24 reps; Eagle Flex I – 2 sets of 22 reps; Bear Flex I – 2 sets of 17 reps; Gorilla Flex I – 2 sets of 17 reps; Elk Flex I – 2 sets of 14 reps (7 Each Arm)

Horse Flex I – 2 sets of 10 reps; Horse Flex II – 2 sets of 15 reps; Horse Flex III – 2 sets of 5 reps; Horse Flex IV – 2 sets of 5 reps; Mule Flex – 2 sets of 5 reps

Tuesday and Friday: Target Muscles → Spine and Neck

Spine: Eel Flex I – 2 sets of 10 reps; Eel Flex II – 2 sets of 10 reps; Alligator Flex I – 2 sets of 15 reps; Alligator Flex II – 2 sets of 10; Eel Flex III – 2 sets of 10 reps

Neck: Bull Flex I – 2 sets of 5 reps; Bull Flex II – 2 sets of 5 reps; Bull Flex III – 2 sets of 10 reps; Giraffe Flex I – 2 sets of 10 reps; Giraffe Flex II – 2 sets of 10 reps

Wednesday and Saturday: Cardiovascular

Elk Climb: 2 sets of 6 reps; Cheetah Dash: 7 reps; Camel Trot: One mile jog;

WEEK 4

Monday & Thursday: Target Muscles → Arms and Abdominal

Gorilla Flex IV – 2 sets of 20 reps; Lion Flex I – 2 sets of 20 reps; Tiger Flex I – 2 sets of 10 reps; Jaguar Flex I – 2 sets 10; Gorilla Flex V – 2 sets of 10 reps

Dolphin Flex I – 2 sets of 30 reps; Dolphin Flex II – 3 sets of 30 reps; Shark Flex I – 2 sets of 20 reps; Shark Flex II – 1 set of 20 reps; Dolphin Flex III – 3 sets of 30 reps

Tuesday & Friday: Target Muscles → Back and Shoulders

Frog Flex I – 4 sets of 20 reps; Frog Flex II – 2 sets of 10 reps; Kangaroo Flex I – 2 sets of 15 reps; Frog Flex III – 2 sets of 10 reps; Kangaroo Flex II – 3 sets of 5 reps each leg

Horse Flex I – 2 sets of 10 reps; Horse Flex II – 2 sets of 15 reps; Horse Flex III – 2 sets of 5 reps; Horse Flex IV – 2 sets of 5 reps; Mule Flex – 2 sets of 5 reps

Wednesday & Saturday: Cardiovascular

Elk Climb: 2 sets of 6 reps; Camel Trot: One mile jog; Cheetah Dash: 8 reps

AN 8-WEEK GET BUFF, GET RIPPED WILDWORKOUT® ROUTINE

Approach: Direct Target, Mix & Match, Circuit

Concentration: TOTAL BODY WORKOUT

Required: Advanced WildWorkout® Training

Caution: For the extremely dedicated only!

Rest Time between sets & exercises for this routine unless otherwise noted is 30 secs-1 minute

Resistance should be 80-100%

WEEK 1

Day 1 & Day 4: Panther Flex I - 20 Reps, 30 Reps, 20 Reps, 30 Reps, Eagle Flex I - 3 Sets of 20 Reps, Bear Flex I - 2 Sets of 20 Reps, Gorilla Flex I - 2 Sets of 20 Reps , Elk Flex I - 2 Sets of 10 reps per side, Dolphin Flex I - 3 Sets of 20 Reps, Dolphin Flex II - 4 Sets of 25 Reps, Shark Flex I - 20 Reps 2 Sets, Shark Flex II - 1 Set 25 Reps, Dolphin Flex III - 4 Sets of 25 Reps

Speed, Energy & Endurance (Direct Target Level 3)

Day 2: Circuit: Panther Flex I - 20 Reps, Dolphin Flex I - 15 Reps, Frog Flex I - 20 Reps, Gorilla Flex I - 10 Reps, Shark Flex I - 10 Reps, Mule Flex - 5 Reps *(Perform Circuit 3 Times)*

Arms (Direct Target Level 3) Shoulders (Direct Target Level 3)

Frog Flex I – 2 Sets of 20 Reps, Frog Flex II – 2 Sets of 10 (Each Part), Kangaroo Flex I – 2 Sets of 10, Frog Flex III – 2 Sets of 10 (Each Leg), Kangaroo Flex II – 2 Sets of 10 (Each position)

Day 3: Back (Direct Target Level 3), Spine (Direct Target Level 3)

Circuit: Bull Flex I - 5 Reps, Bull Flex II - 5 Reps, Bull Flex III - 5 Reps (Each Way), Giraffe Flex I - 5 Reps (Each Way), Giraffe Flex II - 5 Reps (Each Way) *(Perform Circuit 2 Times)*

Camel Trot: Finish Goal=Less than 9 minutes (Rest 2 Minutes), Elk Climb – 2 Sets of 10 Reps, Cheetah Dash 7 Sets of 1 Rep, Camel Trot- WALK- Cool down

Day 4: See Above

Day 5: Panther Flex I - 10 Sets of 10 Reps, Eagle Flex I - 3 Sets of 20 Reps, Bear Flex I - 2 Sets of 20 Reps, Gorilla Flex I - 2 Sets of 20 Reps, Elk Flex I - 2 Sets of 10 reps per side

Abs (Direct Target Level 3 (Sets your choice)), Legs (Frog Flex I & Kangaroo Flex II), Arms (Gorilla Flex IV & Lion Flex I), Shoulders (Direct Target Level 3), Speed, Energy & Endurance (Direct Target Level 3)

Day 6: Back (Direct Target Level 3), Neck (Direct Target Level 3), Spine (Direct Target Level 3), Arms (Mix & Match Pick 3)

Day 7: Rest

WEEK 2

Day 1 & Day 3: Chest (Direct Target Level 3 (Panther Flex I - 4 Sets of 25 Reps), Arms (Direct Target Level 3), Shoulders (Direct Target Level 3), Speed, Energy & Endurance (Level 3)

Day 2: Circuit: Frog Flex I – 25 Reps, Dolphin Flex I – 15 Reps, Elk Climb - 5 Reps, Alligator Flex I – 15 Reps *(Perform Circuit 4 Times)*

Circuit: Dolphin Flex II – 25 Reps, Eel Flex III – 10 Reps, Shark Flex II – 10 Reps (Each Way), Horse Flex I – 10 Reps (Each Side), Alligator Flex II – 10 Reps *(Perform Circuit 4 Times)*

Day 3: See Above

Day 4: Legs (Direct Target Level 3) Abs (Direct Target Level 3) Circuit: Panther Flex I – 10 Reps, Horse Flex IV – 5 Reps, Elk Flex I – 5 Reps (Each Side), Eagle Flex I – 5 Reps *(Perform Circuit 3 Times)*

Day 5: Circuit: Dolphin Flex I – 15 Reps, Dolphin Flex II – 25 Reps, Shark Flex I – 10 Reps, Shark Flex II – 12 Reps (Each Way), Dolphin Flex III – 25 Reps *(Perform Circuit 4 Times)*

Circuit: Panther Flex I – 33 Reps, Eagle Flex I – 20 Reps, Bear Flex I – 10 Reps, Gorilla Flex I – 10 Reps, Elk Flex I – 10 Reps (5 per side) *(Perform Circuit 4 times)* Speed, Energy & Endurance (Direct Target Level 3)

Day 6: Spine & Neck (Direct Target Level 3)

Day 7: Rest

WEEK 3

Day 1: Chest (Direct Target Level 3 (Panther Flex I - 10, 40, 30, 20)), Back (Direct Target Level 3), Circuit: Gorilla Flex III – 10 Reps (Each Arm), Tiger Flex I – 10 Reps (Each Arm) Rhino Flex 1 – 10 Reps (Each Arm), Gorilla Flex V – 5 Reps, Shark Flex I – 15 Reps, Kangaroo Flex II - 5 Reps (Each Way) *(Perform Circuit 3 Times)* Elk Climb 2 Sets of 10 reps

Day 2 & Day 4: Speed, Energy & Endurance (Direct Target Level 3) Frog Flex I- 50 Reps, 30 Reps, 20 Reps, Frog Flex II – 2 Sets of 20 Reps (Each Part)

Day 3: Chest (Direct Target Level 3 (Panther Flex I – 10, 40, 40, 10) Circuit: Shark Flex I - 10 Reps, Dolphin Flex III – 20 Reps, Dolphin Flex I – 15 Reps, Dolphin Flex II – 20 Reps, Shark Flex II – 10 Reps (Each Way) *(Perform Circuit 4 Times)* Circuit: Horse Flex I – 5 Reps (Each Way), Gorilla Flex II – 5 Reps (Each Arm), Horse Flex II – 10 Reps, Gorilla Flex III – 5 Reps (Each Arm), Horse Flex III – 5 Reps, Rhino Flex I – 5 Reps (Each Arm), Horse Flex IV – 5 Reps, Cougar Flex I – 5 Reps (Each Arm), Mule Flex – 5 Reps, Cougar Flex II – 5 Reps (Each Arm) *(Perform Circuit 3 Times)*

Day 4: See Above

Day 5: Circuit: Panther Flex I – 40 Reps, Eagle Flex I – 15 Reps, Kangaroo Flex I – 10 Reps, Frog Flex III – 10 Reps *(Perform Circuit Twice)* Circuit: Dolphin Flex I – 15 Reps, Gorilla Flex IV – 10 Reps (Each Arm- Part One), Shark Flex I – 15 Reps, Lion Flex I – 10 Reps (Each Arm), Shark Flex II – 10 Reps (Each Way) *(Perform Circuit 3 Times)*

Day 6: Circuit: Panther Flex I – 20 Reps, Eagle Flex I – 10 Reps, Bear Flex I – 5 Reps, Gorilla Flex I 5 Reps, Elk Flex I – 5 Reps (5 Each Way) *(Perform Circuit 4 Times)*, Back (Direct Target Level 3), Shoulders (Direct Target Level 3), Cheetah Flex I – 3 Sets of 10 Reps (Each Side), Elk Climb – 2 Sets of 10 Reps, Cheetah Dash – 10 Sets of 1 Rep, Camel Trot, Cheetah Flex II – 2 Sets of 10 Reps

Day 7: Rest

WEEK 4

Day 1, Day 3 & Day 5: Panther Flex I – 50 Reps, Frog Flex I – 50 Reps, Panther Flex 25 Reps, Frog Flex I – 25 Reps, Panther Flex I – 25 Reps, Frog Flex I – 25 Reps, Circuit: Eagle Flex I- 20 Reps, Bear Flex I - 13 Reps, Gorilla Flex I – 13 Reps, Elk Flex -7 Reps (Each Way) *(Perform Circuit 3 Times)* Abdominals (Direct Target Level 3), Speed, Energy & Endurance (Direct Target Level 3)

Day 2: Arms, Back, Shoulders (Direct Target Level 3)

Day 3: See Above

Day 4: Spine, Neck, Arms (Direct Target Level 3)

Day 5: See Above

Day 6: Shoulders, Back, Arms (Direct Target Level 3)

Day 7: Rest

Reminder: Rest Time between sets & exercises for this routine unless otherwise noted is 30 secs-1 minute and Resistance should be 80-100%

WEEK 5

Day 1: Circuit: Panther Flex I – 30 Reps, Alligator Flex I – 15 Reps, Gorilla Flex I – 10 Reps, Alligator Flex II – 10 Reps *(Perform Circuit 3 Times)* Circuit: Dolphin Flex I – 20 Reps, Horse Flex I – 10 Reps (Each Way), Dolphin Flex II – 30 Reps, Horse Flex IV – 5 Reps *(Perform Circuit 3 Times)*, Camel Trot

Day 2: Chest (Direct Target Level 3 (Sets Your Choice)), Arms (Direct Target Level 3), Shoulders (Direct Target Level 3), Speed, Energy & Endurance (Direct Target Level 3)

Day 3: Legs (Direct Target Level 3), Spine (Direct Target Level 3), Neck (Direct Target Level 3), Speed, Energy & Endurance (Direct Target Level 3)

Day 4: Chest (Direct Target Level 3 (Panther Flex 40, 20, 40), Dolphin Flex I – 1 Set 60 Reps, Dolphin Flex II – 2 Sets 50 Reps, Shark Flex I – 1 Set 40 Reps, Shark Flex II – 1 Set 25 Reps (Each Way), Dolphin Flex III, 2 Sets 50 Reps, Camel Trot

Day 5: Arms, Back, Shoulders (Direct Target Level 3)

Day 6: Legs, Shoulders, Spine, (Direct Target Level 3)

Day 7: Rest

WEEK 6

Day 1: Chest (Direct Target Level 3), Abs (Direct Target Level 3), Legs (Direct Target Level 3), Camel Trot

Day 2: Chest (Direct Target Level 3), Arms (Direct Target Level 3), Shoulders (Direct Target Level 3), Cheetah Flex I – 15 Reps (Each Each), Elk Climb 1 Set of 20 Reps

Day 3: Abs (Direct Target Level 3), Legs (Direct Target Level 3), Speed, Energy, & Endurance (Direct Target Level 3)

Day 4: Chest (Direct Target Level 3), Shoulders (Direct Target Level 3), Arms (Direct Target Level 3), Cheetah Flex II – 10 Reps, Cheetah Dash – 10 Reps, Camel Trot

Day 5: Chest, Back, Neck (Direct Target Level 3)

Day 6: Arms, Shoulders, Abdominals (Direct Target Level 3)

Day 7: Rest

WEEK 7

Day 1 & Day 4: Abdominals, Shoulders, Arms (Direct Target Level 3)

Day 2 & Day 5: Legs, Back, Neck (Direct Target Level 3)

Day 3 & Day 6: Chest, Spine, Speed, Energy & Endurance (Direct Target Level 3)

WEEK 8

Day 1: Chest (Direct Target Level 3), Abs, Arms, Shoulders (Mix and Match Pick 2 of each), Speed, Energy & Endurance (Direct Target Level 3)

Day 2: Panther Flex I – 50 Reps, Frog Flex I – 50 Reps, Panther Flex 25 Reps, Frog Flex I – 25 Reps, Panther Flex I – 25 Reps, Frog Flex I – 25 Reps, Back (Direct Target Level 3), Cheetah Flex I – 15 Reps (Each Each), Elk Climb 1 Set of 20 Reps

Day 3: Circuit: Dolphin Flex I – 15 Reps, Dolphin Flex II – 25 Reps, Shark Flex I - 10 Reps, Shark Flex II – 12 Reps (Each Way), Dolphin Flex III – 25 Reps, (Perform Circuit 4 Times), Arms (Direct Target Level 3), Shoulders (Direct Target Level 3)

Day 4: Chest (Direct Target Level 3), Legs (Direct Target Level 3), Spine & Back (Mix and Match Pick 2 Each), Speed, Energy & Endurance (Direct Target Level 3)

Day 5: Chest, Arms, Shoulders (Direct Target Level 3)

Day 6: Abs, Legs, Neck (Direct Target Level 3)

Day 7: Rest

GROUP WORKOUT ROUTINE

Approach Used: Mix & Match

Total Body Workout

Want to exercise with your family, friends, or a group of people?

Try this workout!

Eagle Flex I (2 sets of 10 reps), Bear Flex I (2 sets of 10 reps), Panther Flex I (3 Sets of 10 reps), Frog Flex I (2 sets of 15 reps), Frog Flex III (10 reps per leg), Dolphin Flex I (25 reps), Dolphin Flex II (25 reps), Shark Flex I (15 reps), Shark Flex II (15 reps per side), Eel Flex III (10 reps), Mule Flex (10 Reps), Horse Flex III (10 reps), Alligator Flex I (10 reps), Rhino Flex I (10 reps per side), Gorilla Flex II (10 Reps per side), Cougar Flex I (10 Reps per side), Tiger Flex I (10 Reps per side), Gorilla Flex IV (15 reps per side), Lion Flex I (15 reps per side), Eagle Flex I (10 reps)

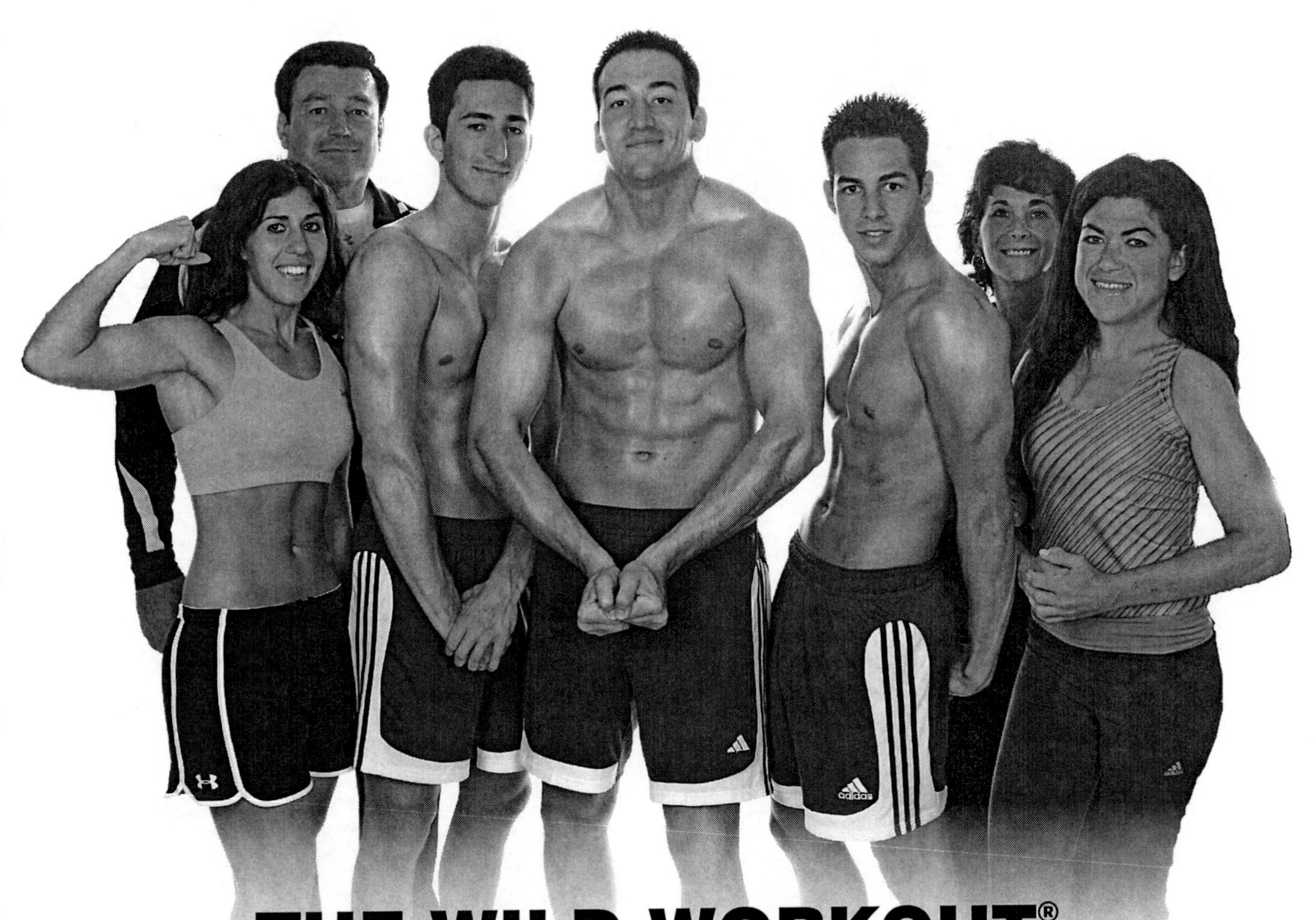

A WORD FROM DR. DWIGHT TAMANAHA

As aholistic consultant and personal trainer and a public speaker on impact-overexertion trauma, I am successfully working with amateur and professional explosive strength athletes. I find the Wild Workout® program to be one of the most effective and powerful ways to build massive amounts of muscle with maximum results in so little time! Building the normally weaker upper body region is crucial for protection against impact-overexertion trauma. The accompaniment of breathing with these exercises pushes oxygen deep into the tissues being exercised.

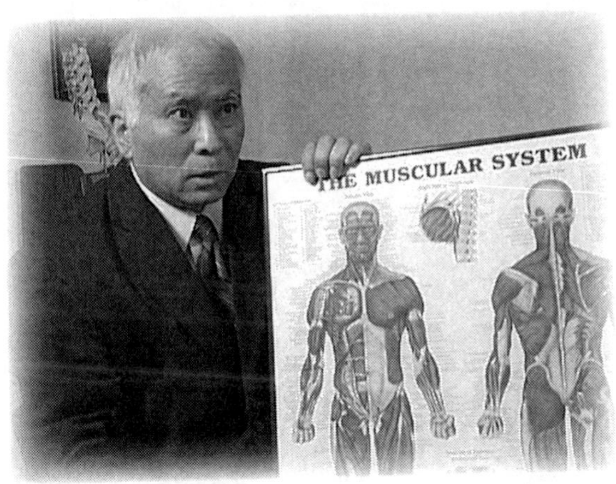

Dr. Dwight Tamanaha

Doctor of Chiropractic
Certified Chiropractic Sports Physician

Dr. Tamanaha is a record-holding Olympic weightlifter in his age and weight class. A former All-American and National Champion, he is published in the Southern Medical Journal, *in a medical textbook, and in the world almanac.*

QUESTIONS & ANSWERS

1. Why do Wild Workout® when I could be lifting weights instead?

Wild Workout® doesn't stress the spine, joints, and connective tissue with added weight, like weightlifting does. Instead, Wild Workout® uses the body's own energy to provide resistance. It turns the body's natural movements—stretching, pulling, pushing, and flexing—into safe, healthful tools for developing strength, flexibility, power and muscle building.

I've been approached by many, many weightlifters who are dealing with chronic physical problems, including deteriorated discs and joints, torn cartilage, torn ligaments, and torn muscles. They've got bad backs, elbows, shoulders, hips, and knees. And unfortunately, many have learned to live with chronic pain.

Early on in a weightlifting workout, the muscles are still fresh enough to do the work of moving the weight. But after a few sets, once the muscles become fatigued, they're less able to support and move the weight. This means the joints, tendons, and ligaments have to do it: a surefire recipe for injury. Over time, heavy weightlifting compresses the spine, squeezing the spinal fluid out of the discs that separate the vertebrae. When there's no padding left to separate the discs, you're left with bone rubbing against bone. And pain.

2. What's the advantage of Wild Workout® over running and other forms of aerobic exercise?

"Aerobic" means "with oxygen," and it's essential that you breathe deeply and regularly while doing your PowerFlexes. Doing this will fill your muscles with the fresh, oxygen-rich blood that muscles need to grow and develop. Actually, all of the PowerFlexes in this course are aerobic.

Sprinting and jogging are excellent. That's why, along with the Cheetah Dash, this course also includes the Camel Trot. However, running alone isn't enough to build complete fitness. And running long distances (longer than five miles) can, over time, cause chronic overuse injuries to the feet, ankles, knees, hips, and back similar to weight lifting problems. People whose only exercise is running long distances, or taking step aerobics or "spinning" classes, usually look healthy when they're fully clothed but since their routines don't include muscle building exercises, they may have skinny arms, narrow shoulders, and sunken chests. Maybe even flabby abs.

If you run long distances, you owe it to your long-term health to supplement your running with a low-impact, joint-friendly strength training program such as Wild Workout®.

3. Why do Wild Workout® instead of working out at a gym or a health/fitness club?

With clubs and gyms, you're paying constantly—to be taught how to use the exercise equipment, then to continue to use it. You pay for that equipment to be maintained and sanitized regularly. And for all the extras, such as juice bars and cable TV, whether you use or want them or not. If you've got a tight schedule, working out at a health club means finding time to drive to the club, paying for gas to get there and back, find a parking place, change clothes, and stand in line to use the equipment—whether the equipment has been sanitized or not.

This Wild Workout® course provides much better value for your money. It's like an owner's manual for the human body, showing you how to use your own energy and ability to sculpt your muscles, build strength, health, and add power. You can PowerFlex® wherever you are, whenever it's convenient. You can listen to your favorite music or watch your favorite TV show. You only pay for it once, your investment will pay for itself over and over again.

4. Why PowerFlex® instead of using one of those home gym machines?

Consider the cost. Many of those treadmills, machines, gadgets, equipment and weights cost hundreds—or thousands—of dollars. And once the maintenance contract runs out—if you bought one—repair bills add to your cost.

Exercise machines are not only expensive, but they can be dangerous, too. Seats and pins break, benches collapse, and bands snap—sometimes causing serious injuries.

Thousands of these contraptions have been recalled by their manufacturers due to mechanical breakdowns (and lawsuits). On TV they always work perfectly and take up minimal floor space. But once they're delivered and set up, they're often bigger than they appear on TV. And more difficult to use. All these reasons explain why so many exercise machines become big, expensive racks to hang your old clothes on, and why so many owners give up and try to sell them, hoping to get back even a fraction of their investment.

Wild Workout® is a far better value. You're paying for a lifetime of fitness, not for big, expensive, complicated gadgets. You only pay for it once, and it's as portable as you are. You can PowerFlex® whenever it's convenient. And best of all, Wild Workout® teaches you how to get the most out of the most brilliantly designed, incredibly functional machine you'll ever use: your own body.

5. How fit do I have to be before I can do Wild Workout®?

Whether you're already fit or have never exercised in your life, Wild Workout® lets you start where you are and will get you to your fitness goals, whatever they are. In no time at all you can build huge, bulging muscles and massive strength, like a gorilla, or lean, sculpted muscles with explosive power, like a panther. The more resistance you use and the higher the number of repetitions you do, the bigger your muscles will grow. With Wild Workout® achieving your fitness goals will be easy.

6. What makes Wild Workout® better than other exercise or fitness courses?

Wild Workout® covers every muscle in your body from head to toe and nothing is left up to guess work. Wild Workout® tell you what exercises to do, how many exercises to do, and how to do the exercises to get the body of your dreams there is no guess work or confusion. It also gives to you the ability to become your own best personal trainer, teaching you how to mix and match the PowerFlexes to build, sculpt, and shape your muscles and also shows you how to target your problem areas that you have in your body which you never knew how to deal with to get the results that you never thought possible.

With the 45 PowerFlexes to choose from you have such a variety that you can build completely different full body workouts of your own and never do the same routine twice, boredom from doing the same old routines are never an issue. It is truly amazing and it works, it's the Real Deal, No bull, No hype! It is all accomplished with no weights, no pulleys, no bars, no bands, no machines, no equipment, no drugs, no steroids, and no pills. It is the real deal No ifs ands or buts! You might say "but my friend says..., but my coach says..., but my brother says..." No, you get your BUT out of the way, do this workout and you will see results that nobody can talk you out of! Don't let anybody hinder you from getting the Body you want!

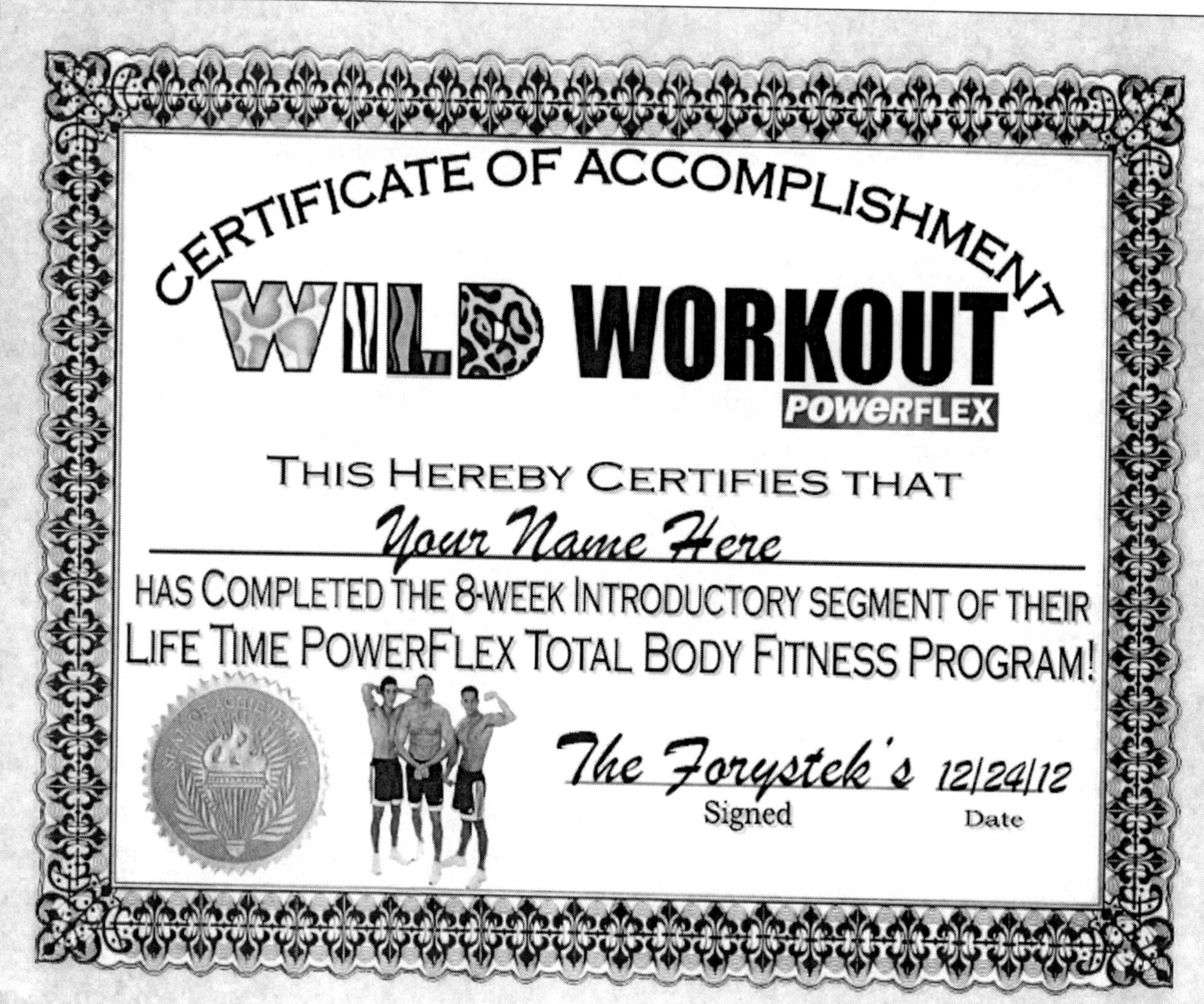
CERTIFICATE OF ACCOMPLISHMENT
WILD WORKOUT
POWERFLEX
THIS HEREBY CERTIFIES THAT
Your Name Here
HAS COMPLETED THE 8-WEEK INTRODUCTORY SEGMENT OF THEIR
LIFE TIME POWERFLEX TOTAL BODY FITNESS PROGRAM!
The Forystek's
Signed
12/24/12
Date

CERTIFICATE OF ACCOMPLISHMENT

Receive your very own Beautiful Suitable for framing Wild Workout® diploma! Celebrate your great fitness achievement. You will want to display this beautiful diploma for all to see! You are serious about health and fitness and we would like to acknowledge your dedication.

Send a Self-Addressed Stamped Envelope to:
Forystek Fitness Corp.
P. O. Box 28403
Green Bay, WI 54324

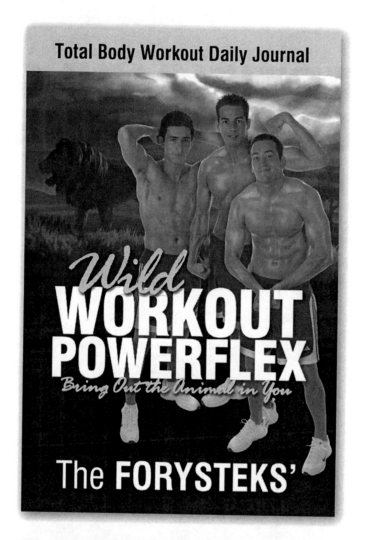

POWERFLEX®

Order your PowerFlex® Journal and DVD online at
www.TheWildWorkout.com
products page and we will ship it out to you immediately.

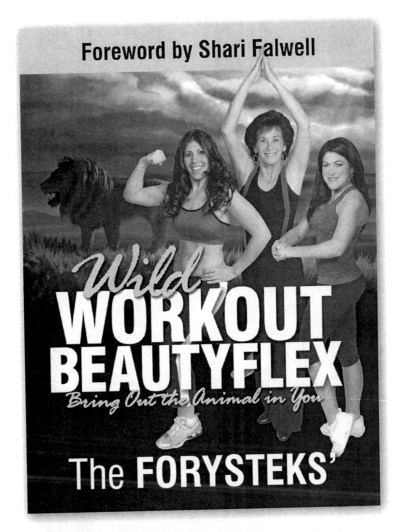

BEAUTYFLEX®

Order your BeautyFlex® Workbook, Journal and DVD online at
www.TheWildWorkout.com
products page and we will ship it out to you immediately.

CPSIA information can be obtained
at www.ICGtesting.com
Printed in the USA
FFOW01n1227260515
13576FF